MCQs for the FRCS(Urol) and Postgraduate Urology Examinations

MCQs for the FRCS(Urol) and Postgraduate Urology Examinations

Edited by

Manit Arya
MBChB, FRCS, MD(Res), FRCS(Urol)

Taimur T. Shah
MBBS, BSc(Hons), FRCS(Urol)

Jas S. Kalsi
MBBS, BSc(Hons), MD(Res), MRCS(Eng), FRCS(Urol)

Herman S. Fernando
MBBS, MS, DNB, MRCSEd, MD, FRCS(Urol), FEBU

Iqbal S. Shergill
MBBS, BSc(Hons), MRCS, FRCS(Urol), FEBU

Asif Muneer
BSc(Hons), MBChB, MD, FRCSEd, FRCS(Urol)

Hashim U. Ahmed
FRCS(Urol), PhD, BM, BCh, MA

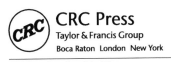

CRC Press
Taylor & Francis Group
Boca Raton London New York

CRC Press is an imprint of the
Taylor & Francis Group, an **informa** business

First edition published 2020
by CRC Press
6000 Broken Sound Parkway NW, Suite 300, Boca Raton, FL 33487-2742

and by CRC Press
2 Park Square, Milton Park, Abingdon, Oxon, OX14 4RN

© 2020 Taylor & Francis Group, LLC

CRC Press is an imprint of Taylor & Francis Group, LLC

Library of Congress Cataloging-in-Publication Data

Names: Arya, M. (Manit), editor.
Title: MCQs for the FRCS(Urol) and postgraduate urology examinations /
    edited by Manit Arya [and six others].
Description: First edition. | Boca Raton : CRC Press, 2020. | Includes
    bibliographical references and index. | Summary: "This book provides a
    selection of representative MCQs together with a detailed explanation of
    each answer covering the topic in depth. Each chapter has been written
    by experienced Urological surgeons who have already been successful in
    passing the examination. In addition to the FRCS(Urol) examination MCQs
    form the basis of equivalent postgraduate Urological examinations
    internationally and the scope of this book will be an invaluable
    addition to individuals sitting the FEBU and similar exams in the USA,
    Australia and Asian countries. Established consultants may also find the
    text useful as a 'refresher' in areas outside their subspecialist
    interest"-- Provided by publisher.
Identifiers: LCCN 2020004716 (print) | LCCN 2020004717 (ebook) | ISBN
    9780367076184 (paperback) | ISBN 9780429021633 (ebook)
Subjects: MESH: Urologic Diseases | Urogenital Neoplasms | Examination
    Questions
Classification: LCC RC871 (print) | LCC RC871 (ebook) | NLM WJ 18.2 |
    DDC 616.60076--dc23
LC record available at https://lccn.loc.gov/2020004716
LC ebook record available at https://lccn.loc.gov/2020004717

ISBN: 9780367076184 (pbk)
ISBN: 9780429021633 (ebk)

Typeset in Rotis
by Lumina Datamatics Limited

Contents

Editors

Manit Arya is a Consultant Urological Surgeon at Imperial College NHS Trust London (Charing Cross Hospital) and University College Hospital, London. His research interests include investigating the molecular basis of prostate cancer – he has been awarded a MD Higher Research degree from the University of London in this field. He has published extensively in peer-reviewed journals particularly in the field of prostate cancer and is an editor of 10 text-books. He is a Principal Investigator of several National Clinical Trials involving focal therapies (cryotherapy and HIFU) for prostate cancer.

Taimur T. Shah is a final year trainee in London who has a sub-specialist interest in imaging, focal and radical therapy for prostate cancer and is involved in clinical trials for primary, meta-static and radio-recurrent prostate cancer. He is a member of the Imperial Prostate (IP) Research Group at Imperial College London (ICL) and also vice chair of the British Urology Researchers in Surgical Training (BURST) research collaborative.

Jas S. Kalsi is a Consultant Urological Surgeon and Andrologist at Imperial College in London and at Frimley Health in Surrey and Berkshire. He runs a regional andrology service based at Charing Cross Hospital and at Wexham Park. He is currently a clinical lead and clinical governance lead at Wexham Park and Heatherwood Hospitals. He is actively involved in education and is a national trainer for holmium laser enucleation of the prostate (HoLEP) in the UK. He has been a Foundation Training Programme director and educational supervisor for 5 years for the Oxford Deanery. He is a member of the urology STC in North Thames. He is on the Trust patient safety and consent committee and has a commitment to patient safety and governance. His main clinical interests include andrology (Peyronie's disease, male factor infertility and severe ED) and the management of large and complex benign prostates including HoLEP surgery.

Herman S. Fernando is a Consultant Urological Surgeon at University Hospital of North Midlands NHS Trust and an Honorary Clinical Lecturer at Keele University. He was trained as a Surgeon in India and subsequently did basic science research on prostate cancer at Cardiff University. He has published papers in high impact journals and is actively involved in teaching, assessments, standard setting and examinations for various regional and national institutions. He is the winner of the BAUS Silver Cystoscope award for the Best Trainer in UK in 2019. His main clinical areas of interest are Robotic/Laparoscopic Upper Tract Oncology and Stone Diseases.

Iqbal S. Shergill is a Consultant Urological Surgeon in Wrexham Maelor Hospital, Betsi Cadwaladr University Health Board, Wales; Professor of Urological Innovation at Glyndwr University, Wrexham and Clinical Director of the North Wales Clinical Research Centre, Wrexham; Honorary Senior Lecturer at Manchester Medical School, The University of Manchester; Honorary Senior Lecturer in the Division of Biological Sciences, University of Chester; Honorary Senior Lecturer in the Division of Medical Sciences, Bangor University; and Honorary Clinical Teacher at Cardiff University School of Medicine, Wales. He has an active interest in teaching, education and research. He has been an Assigned Educational Supervisor for Urology trainees, Lecturer on Core Urology Course, Panellist at National Selection for Urology Training and is currently Course Director of Rapid Revision Course for FRCS(Urol). He has been on the Executive Committee for Academic Urology (BAUS) and Clinical Director at the North Wales and North West Urological Research Centre.

Asif Muneer is a Consultant Urological Surgeon and Andrologist based at University College London Hospital, UK and Hon Associate Professor at UCL. Having completed his medical degree (MD) at UCL, he went on to higher surgical training in Oxford. He has published widely on all aspects of urology with his main interest in andrology and has also edited the *Textbook of Penile*

Cancer, Atlas of Male Genitourethral Surgery and *Prosthetic Surgery in Urology*. He has lectured both nationally and internationally and is the Past President of the British Society for Sexual Medicine and the Ex Chair of the BAUS Section of Andrology. He is the current Hon Secretary of BAUS.

Hashim U. Ahmed is Chair of Urology at Imperial College London. Hashim is an internationally renowned expert in prostate cancer diagnosis, imaging and biopsy as well as minimally invasive therapies for prostate cancer. He has taught dozens of surgeons in these techniques in the UK and around the world and given numerous invited international lectures in this area as well as Visiting Professor at a number of institutions. He majors in methodological research in imaging and surgical methods and has an extensive research portfolio with about £6M in grant income as a principal applicant and co-applicant to a research programme of approximately £14M. He has published over 150 peer-reviewed papers in areas that have led to key changes in the way we diagnose and treat men with localised prostate cancer.

Contributors

Hamid Abboudi
Charing Cross Hospital
Imperial College Healthcare NHS Trust
London, United Kingdom

Mohamed Yehia Abdallah
Wrexham Maelor Hospital
Betsi Cadwaladr University Health Board
North Wales, United Kingdom

Sanjay Agarwal
Wrexham Maelor Hospital
Wrexham, United Kingdom

Vineet Agrawal
Urology
The Guthrie Clinic
Sayre, Pennsylvania

Hashim U. Ahmed
Department of Surgery and Cancer
Imperial College
and
Imperial Urology
Imperial College Healthcare NHS Trust
London, United Kingdom

Tev Aho
Addenbrooke's Hospital
Cambridge, United Kingdom

Adam Alleemudder
King George Hospital
Barking, Havering and Redbridge University
    Hospitals NHS Trust
Ilford, United Kingdom

Hussain M. Alnajjar
University College London Hospital NHS
    Trust
London, United Kingdom

James Armitage
Addenbrooke's Hospital
Cambridge, United Kingdom

Manit Arya
Imperial College Healthcare NHS Trust
University College Hospital
London, United Kingdom

Nish Bedi
Specialist Registrar
North Thames, United Kingdom

Simon R. J. Bott
Frimley Park Hospital
Camberley, United Kingdom

Noel Clarke
Christie Hospital
Christie NHS Hospital Foundation Trust
Manchester, United Kingdom

Paul Cleaveland
The Christie NHS Foundation Trust
Manchester, United Kingdom

Angela Cottrell
Royal Devon & Exeter Hospital
Exeter, United Kingdom

David Cranston
Oxford University Hospitals NHS Foundation
    Trust
Oxford, United Kingdom

Amr Emara
Frimley Park Hospital
Camberley, United Kingdom

Herman S. Fernando
University Hospital of North Midlands NHS
    Trust
Stoke-on-Trent, United Kingdom

Lyndon Gommersall
University Hospital of North Midlands NHS Trust
Stoke on Trent, United Kingdom

Anuj Goyal
Barnet and Chase Farm Hospitals NHS Trust
Enfield, United Kingdom

Jemma Hale
Kent and Canterbury Hospital
East Kent Hospitals University NHS Foundation
    Trust
Kent, United Kingdom

Rizwan Hamid
University College Hospital
London, United Kingdom

Hashim Hashim
Urology
Bristol Urological Institute
Bristol, United Kingdom

Beth Hickerton
Royal Liverpool and Broadgreen University
    Hospitals NHS Trust
Liverpool, United Kingdom

Rozh Jalil
Kings College Hospital NHS Foundation Trust
London, United Kingdom

Thomas Johnston
Norfolk and Norwich University Hospital
Norwich, United Kingdom

Jas S. Kalsi
Frimley Health NHS Foundation Trust
Frimley, United Kingdom

Farooq Khan
Luton and Dunstable University Hospital NHS
    Foundation Trust
Luton, United Kingdom

David Mak
Royal Wolverhampton NHS Trust
Wolverhampton, United Kingdom

David A. Manson-Bahr
The Royal Marsden NHS Foundation Trust
London, United Kingdom

Shyam Matanhelia
Royal Blackburn Hospital
Blackburn, United Kingdom

Erik Mayer
Department of Surgery & Cancer
Imperial College London
London, United Kingdom

Asif Muneer
University College London Hospital NHS Trust
and
NIHR Biomedical Research Centre
University College London Hospitals
and
Division of Surgery and Interventional Science
University College London
London, United Kingdom

Vinodh Murali
Mujilibhai Patel Urological Hospital
Nadiad, India
and
University Hospital of North Midlands NHS
    Trust
Stoke-on-Trent, United Kingdom

Nkwam Nkwam
King's College Hospital NHS Foundation
    Trust
London, United Kingdom

Ali Omar
Wexham Park Hospital
Slough, United Kingdom

Nilay Patel (deceased)
Churchill Hospital
Oxford, United Kingdom

Tina Rashid
Imperial College Healthcare NHS Trust
London, United Kingdom

Vijay Sangar
Christie Hospital
Christie NHS Hospital Foundation Trust
Manchester, United Kingdom

Taimur T. Shah
London NHS
Imperial College London
London, United Kingdom

Davendra M. Sharma
St Georges Hospital
London, United Kingdom

Iqbal S. Shergill
Wrexham Maelor Hospital
Betsi Cadwaladr University Health Board
North Wales, United Kingdom

Chitranjan J. Shukla
Western General Hospital
Edinburgh, United Kingdom

Arash K. Taghizadeh
Evelina Children's Hospital
London, United Kingdom

Ali Tasleem
Princess Royal University Hospital
Orpington, United Kingdom

Rebecca Tregunna
University Hospitals of North Midlands NHS
    Trust
London, United Kingdom

Justin Vale
Department of Surgery & Cancer
Imperial College London
London, United Kingdom

Oliver Wiseman
Addenbrooke's Hospital
Cambridge, United Kingdom

Introduction

This book is unique in that it is the first MCQ revision book to be published specifically for candidates sitting the FRCS(Urol) examination. Together with the published and companion book *Viva Practice for the FRCS(Urol) and Postgraduate Urology Examinations*, it will form the basis of the well-established course titled 'Rapid Revision for the FRCS(Urol)' (this course is run by the editors of both books).

The FRCS(Urol) examination is set to test the required standard of a recognised Urology specialist in the UK (i.e., a day one NHS UK/Ireland consultant). The examination is divided into two parts. The first part is devoted entirely to MCQs that aim to test the entire urology syllabus in depth.

The second part uses clinical scenarios to form the basis of the *viva voce* section of the examination. These vivas test the candidate on the domains of overall professional capability, knowledge and judgement, logical thought process, safe practice and communication skills.

The aim of this book is to provide a selection of representative MCQs together with a detailed explanation of each answer covering the topic in depth. Each chapter has been written by experienced Urological surgeons who have already been successful in passing the examination.

In addition to the FRCS(Urol) examination MCQs form the basis of equivalent postgraduate Urological examinations internationally and the scope of this book will be an invaluable addition to individuals sitting the FEBU and similar exams in the USA, Australia and Asian countries. Established consultants may also find the text useful as a 'refresher' in areas outside their subspecialist interest.

Manit Arya
Taimur T. Shah
Jas S. Kalsi
Herman S. Fernando
Iqbal S. Shergill
Asif Muneer
Hashim U. Ahmed

CHAPTER 1: ANATOMY & EMBRYOLOGY

Ali Tasleem and Adam Alleemudder

MCQs

Q1. Anatomy of the ureter. Which one is TRUE?
- A. Along its course, the ureter passes in front of the gonadal vessels and behind the bifurcation of the common iliac vessels.
- B. The wall of the ureter has three layers.
- C. The ureter originates in front of the renal artery.
- D. The blood supply to the ureter includes the middle rectal artery.
- E. There are two areas of narrowing along the length of the ureter.

Q2. Anatomy of the renal vasculature. Which one is TRUE?
- A. The posterior segmental artery is formed after entering the renal hilum.
- B. Arcuate arteries give rise to interlobar arteries.
- C. There are four anterior segmental arteries.
- D. PUJ obstruction may be caused by an anterior segmental artery.
- E. The left renal vein passes in front of the superior mesenteric artery to reach the IVC.

Q3. Which one of the following is TRUE regarding the adrenal glands?
- A. The right gland is round in shape and lies lower than the left.
- B. The zona fasciculata produces sex hormones.
- C. The cortex contains chromaffin cells, which produce catecholamines.
- D. The blood supply to the adrenal gland includes the inferior phrenic artery.
- E. Postganglionic sympathetic fibres directly innervate the adrenal glands.

Q4. Anatomy of the penis. Which one of the following is TRUE?
- A. The corpus spongiosum is attached to the inferior ischiopubic rami at the root of the penis.
- B. The cavernosal artery supplies the urethra, glans and spongiosum.
- C. Buck's fascia is continuous with Colles' fascia in the perineum.
- D. The cavernosal nerve provides sensory supply to the penile skin.
- E. The arcuate subpubic ligament helps to maintain the erect penis in an upright position.

Q5. Anatomy of the anterior abdominal wall and fascial layers. Which one of the following is TRUE?
- A. The aponeuroses all pass in front of the rectus muscle at the level of the umbilicus.
- B. Pyramidalis muscle acts to stabilise the linea alba and keep it taut.
- C. The internal oblique originates from the anterior aspect of the lower eight ribs.
- D. The deep inguinal ring is medial to the inferior epigastric artery.
- E. Camper's fascia lines the scrotum and perineum.

Q6. Embryology of the gonads. Which one of the following is TRUE?
- A. The genital ridges develop during the 12th week.
- B. In female embryos, Müllerian Inhibiting Substance causes regression of the paramesonephric duct.
- C. Sertoli cells secrete testosterone that plays a role in embryogenesis.
- D. Hydatid of Morgagni is a remnant of the paramesonephric duct.
- E. The testes reach the inguinal region by the 24th week.

Q7. Anatomy of the kidneys. Which one of the following is TRUE?
A. The left kidney lies between L1 and L3.
B. The dromedary hump on the medial aspect of the kidney is more common on the right.
C. The lower pole of the kidney is more medial and posterior than the upper pole.
D. Gerota's fascia surrounds the kidney except medially where there is a potential open space.
E. The main lymphatic drainage from the left kidney is into the lateral paraaortic nodes.

Q8. Which of the following is TRUE regarding the prostate?
A. The prostate gland develops from the distal nephric ducts.
B. The majority of cancers originate from the central zone.
C. Fibromuscular stroma makes up 70% of the prostate.
D. The blood supply to the prostate is from the pudendal artery.
E. The glandular elements drain into the urethra at the verumontanum.

Q9. Regarding the bladder, which of the following is FALSE?
A. The urachus is the remnant of the allantois.
B. During filling, the bladder neck rises upwards.
C. The ureters are surrounded by the Sheath of Waldeyer.
D. The middle circular and outer longitudinal fibres are deficient around the bladder neck in women.
E. The urothelium overlying the trigone is thinnest.

Q10. Regarding the urethra, which of the following is TRUE?
A. Transitional cell epithelium lines the length of the urethra.
B. The external urethral sphincter is supplied by the cavernosal nerve.
C. Bulbourethral glands open into the membranous urethra.
D. The external sphincter completely surrounds the urethra in women.
E. Skene glands release mucus into the vestibule in women.

EMQs

Q11. Anatomy of the female organs
1. Infundibulum of uterine tube
2. Ampulla of uterine tube
3. Broad ligament
4. Round ligament
5. Mesovarium ligament
6. Suspensory ligament
7. Uterine artery
8. Ovarian artery
9. Vaginal artery
10. Cardinal ligament

For each of the descriptions below, choose the most appropriate structure from the list above.

A. Site of fertilisation of the ovum
B. Connects the uterus to the pelvic side wall
C. Attaches the ovary to the broad ligament
D. Attaches the ovary to the pelvic wall
E. Attaches the ovary to the uterus
F. Surrounded by fimbriae
G. Branch of the internal iliac artery
H. Runs in the suspensory ligament
I. Branches also supply the fallopian tubes
J. Connects the cervix with the lateral pelvic wall

Q12. Embryology of the urinary system

1. Pronephros
2. Mesonephros
3. Metanephros
4. Cloaca
5. Mesonephric duct
6. Seminal vesicles
7. Intermediate mesoderm
8. Nephrogenic cord
9. Ureteric bud
10. Urogenital sinus
11. Paramesonephric duct

For each of the descriptions below, choose the most appropriate structure from the list above.

A. Temporary functional unit that regresses by the 8th week of gestation
B. Non-functioning unit that develops in the 3rd week of gestation
C. Becomes the definitive kidney
D. Unsegmented intermediate mesoderm
E. Develops adjacent to the nephrogenic cord during the 4th week
F. Common mesodermal ridge that gives rise to the three overlapping kidney structures
G. Arises from the mesonephric duct to give rise to the renal pelvis and calyces
H. Drains urine from the intermediate mesoderm and mesonephric duct
I. Forms from the mesonephric duct
J. Embryological origin of the bladder and urethra
K. Becomes the uterus, fallopian tubes and upper two-thirds of the vagina

Q13. Anatomy of the pelvis and perineum.

1. False pelvis
2. True pelvis
3. Obturator nerve
4. Sacrotuberous and sacrospinous
5. Obturator internus
6. Levator ani and coccygeus
7. Puborectalis
8. Perineal body
9. Urogenital hiatus
10. Superficial perineal pouch

For each of the descriptions below, choose the most appropriate structure from the list above.

A. Provides sensation to the medial aspect of the upper thigh and motor innervations to the adductors of the leg
B. Divides the sciatic foramen into lesser and greater parts
C. Root of penis originates from this area
D. Allows the urethra to pass through the pelvic floor
E. Bounded by the lumbar vertebrae, iliacus and anterior abdominal wall
F. Forms the pelvic floor
G. Passes through the lesser sciatic foramen and attaches to the femur
H. Bounded by pubic symphysis, iliopectineal lines and sacral promontory
I. Focal attachment point for the pelvic floor muscles and fascia
J. Forms part of levator ani

Q14. Anatomy of the nervous system.

1. Somatic nervous system
2. Autonomic nervous system
3. Superior hypogastric plexus
4. Somatic lumbosacral plexus
5. Iliohypogastric nerve
6. Obturator nerve
7. Ilioinguinal nerve
8. Femoral nerve
9. Genitofemoral nerve
10. Lateral cutaneous nerve of the thigh

For each of the descriptions below, choose the most appropriate structure from the list above.

A. Superior branch of the anterior rami of L1
B. Disruption causes retrograde ejaculation
C. Passes under the inguinal ligament to supply quadriceps
D. Involved in the cremasteric reflex
E. Provides sensation to the anterior scrotum
F. Originates from the anterior rami of L2 to L3
G. Supplies smooth muscle
H. Provides sensory innervations to medial aspect of thigh
I. Supplies skeletal muscle
J. Originate from L1 to S3

Q15. Great vessels
1. Inferior phrenic artery
2. Celiac trunk
3. Renal artery
4. Middle sacral
5. External iliac artery
6. Accessory obturator artery
7. Internal pudendal artery
8. Umbilical artery
9. Left adrenal vein
10. Posterior trunk of internal iliac artery

For each of the descriptions below, choose the most appropriate structure from the list above.

A. Branch from the aorta at the level of L2
B. Gives off the deep circumflex iliac and inferior epigastric arteries
C. Gives rise to the superior vesical artery
D. First branch of the abdominal aorta
E. Drains into the renal vein
F. Found in 25% of individuals
G. Gives rise to the common hepatic artery
H. Final branch of the aorta
I. Gives off the iliolumbar artery
J. Leaves through the greater sciatic foramen and then re-enters through the lesser sciatic foramen

MCQs – ANSWERS

Q1. Answer D

The ureter is up to 30 cm long. From its origin behind the renal artery, each ureter descends over the anterior border of the psoas to the pelvis. In doing so, it passes behind the gonadal vessels but over the bifurcation of the common iliac vessels. In men, the ureter continues along the lateral wall of the pelvis and then turns forward at the ischial spine to enter the bladder just after it is crossed by the vas deferens. In women, the ureter turns forwards and medially at the ischial spine and runs in the base of the broad ligament where it is crossed by the uterine artery. It continues forward passing the lateral fornix of the vagina to enter the bladder. The **four** layers in the wall of the ureter include the inner transitional cell epithelium, lamina propria, smooth muscle and outer adventitia. The blood supply is from several sources; in the abdomen the ureter receives branches from the renal, gonadal, common iliac arteries and the abdominal aorta. In the pelvis, it is supplied by the internal iliac artery and its branches including the vesicle, uterine, vaginal and middle rectal arteries. There are three main points of narrowing along its course: at the pelvi-ureteric and vesico-ureteric junctions and over the common iliac vessels.

Q2. Answer C

Roughly a quarter of the cardiac output is supplied to the kidneys via the paired renal arteries. They branch from the aorta at the level of L2 just below the origins of the superior mesenteric (SMA) and adrenal arteries. The right artery passes behind the inferior vena cava (IVC) first, in contrast to the left, which passes almost directly to the kidney. Before entering the hilum, each artery initially gives off a single **posterior segmental branch** that passes behind the renal pelvis to supply the posterior aspect of the kidney. It can cause obstruction of the pelvi-ureteric junction if it passes in front of the ureter. After entering the hilum, the artery commonly divides into four **anterior segmental branches** (apical, upper, middle and lower). The divisions and blood supply of the anterior and posterior segmental arteries give rise to a longitudinal avascular plane, known as Brodel's line, 1–2 cm posterior to convex border of the kidney. Segmental arteries give rise to **lobar arteries** within the renal sinus, which become **interlobar arteries** that lie in between the Columns of Bertin in the parenchyma. These give off **arcuate branches**, which become the **interlobular arteries** that eventually form the **afferent arteries** of the glomeruli. The renal vein lies in front of the artery in the renal hilum. The right vein is 2–4 cm in length in comparison to the left, which may be up to 10 cm. The left renal vein reaches the IVC by passing behind the SMA and in most cases in front of the aorta.

Q3. Answer D

The pair of adrenal glands are located just above each kidney in the retroperitoneum enclosed by Gerota's fascia. In the newborn, the glands weigh much more but the cortex undergoes a degree of atrophy over the following 12 months to reach the adult weight of 5 g. The right gland is more triangular in shape and lies higher than the left. Each is made up of an outer **cortex** and an inner **medulla**, which contains catecholamine producing chromaffin cells. The cortex makes up the majority of the gland weight and consists of three distinct zones producing different hormones:

- Outer **zona glomerulosa** – Mineralocorticoids (e.g., aldosterone)
- Middle **zona fasciculata** – Glucocorticoids (e.g., cortisol)
- Inner **zona reticularis** – Sex hormones

The blood supplying the glands stems from the aorta, inferior phrenic and ipsilateral renal arteries. Preganglionic sympathetic fibres directly innervate the medulla to stimulate catecholamine release.

Q4. Answer E

The two **corpora cavernosa** originate as the crus penis from the inferior ischiopubic rami and perineal membrane in the superficial pouch. Their outer surfaces are covered by the ischicavernosus muscles. They come together below the pubic symphysis, separated by a midline septum and surrounded by the tunica albuginea. The **corpus spongiosum** lies underneath in a groove and contains the urethra. The proximal end is dilated to form the bulb of the penis, which originates from the centre of the perineal membrane, and is covered by the bulbospongiosus muscle. Distally, the spongiosum expands and caps the two corpora to form the glans penis, containing the external urethral meatus at its tip. The three bodies are further surrounded by a deeper Buck's fascia, which merges proximally with the tunica albuginea, and a superficial dartos fascia, which merges with Colles' fascia in the perineum. The suspensory ligament helps to maintain the erect penis in an upright position for coitus and has three components including, the **superficial fundiform, suspensory ligament proper** and the **arcuate subpubic ligaments**. The penis and urethra is supplied by the **internal pudendal artery**, which divides into three branches:

- **Bulbourethral** – Supplies the urethra, spongiosum and glans penis.
- **Cavernosal** – Passes through the middle of each cavernosa to supply the sinuses.
- **Dorsal artery of penis** – Passes underneath Buck's fascia towards the glans to supply the spongiosum and urethra.

The skin and dorsal structures are supplied by the **external pudendal artery**, which runs in the dartos fascia and originates from the femoral artery.

The nerves supplying the penis include:

- **Dorsal** – Passes underneath Buck's fascia to supply the glans penis.
- **Cavernosal** – Provides autonomic supply to the corporal bodies.
- **Perineal** – Supplies the ventral aspect of the penis.

Q5. Answer B

The anterior abdominal wall is made up of several layers including skin, superficial (Camper's) and deep (Scarpa's) fascia, muscle, extraperitoneal fascia and parietal peritoneum. **Camper's fascia** is just beneath the skin and continuous with the superficial fat over the rest of the body. **Scarpa's fascia** blends with the superficial layer superiorly and laterally but inferiorly it continues as the deep fascia of the thigh 1 cm below the inguinal ligament, and medially, it becomes **Buck's fascia**. **Colles' fascia** lines the scrotum (or labia majora) and perineum and inserts posteriorly to the edges of the urogenital diaphragm and inferior ischiopubic rami. The wall musculature consists of the outer **external oblique, internal oblique** and inner **transversus abdominus**. They play a role in respiration, movement and increase abdominal pressure during micturition, defaecation and childbirth. The external oblique originates from the anterior surface of the lower 8th rib and inserts inferiorly to the lateral half of the iliac crest and medially to the rectus sheath. Its fibres run lateral to medial. The internal oblique originates from the lumbodorsal fascia and iliac crest. Its fibres run at right angles to the external oblique, from medial to lateral, and the muscle inserts onto the anterior surface of the lower four ribs and the rectus sheath medially. Transversus abdominis originates from the lumbodorsal fascia and iliac crest and inserts medially into the rectus sheath. Its fibres run horizontally. The aponeuroses of the three muscles form the rectus sheath that surrounds the rectus abdominis muscle and they meet in the midline to form the avascular **linea alba**. The composition of the rectus sheath varies depending on the arbitrary **arcuate line**, which is a third of the way from the umbilicus to the pubic symphysis. Below the line, the aponeuroses of all three muscles pass in front of the rectus abdominis, leaving its posterior surface covered by transversalis fascia. Above the line, the rectus is covered anteriorly by the aponeuroses of the external and internal oblique, and posteriorly by the aponeuroses of internal oblique and transversus abdominis. The sheath is attached to the rectus abdominis anteriorly at segmental tendinous intersections. **Pyramidalis**, when present, lies in front of the lower end of rectus abdominis that originates from the pubic symphysis and inserts into the linea alba. The **inguinal canal** lies parallel to and just above the inguinal ligament at the lower end of the anterior abdominal wall that transmits the ilioingui-nal nerve and the spermatic cord (round ligament in women). It is 4 cm in length and extends medially and inferiorly from the deep (internal) to the superficial (external) inguinal rings. The boundaries of the canal include the inguinal ligament in the floor, the external oblique as the anterior wall (reinforced laterally by the internal oblique), mainly tranversalis fascia as the back wall and the roof by the conjoint tendon, which is formed from fusion of the lower fibres of internal oblique and transversus abdominis. The **deep ring** is an opening in the transversalis fascia that lies 1 cm above the inguinal ligament midway between the anterior superior iliac spine and pubic symphysis. The **inferior epigastric artery** lies medial to the ring. The **super-ficial ring** lies medial to and above the pubic tubercle and is an opening within the external oblique aponeurosis. The upper abdominal wall is supplied by the superior epigastric artery (branch of the internal thoracic artery) and the lower half by the deep circumflex iliac and inferior epigastric arteries (branches of the external iliac artery).

Q6. Answer D

The sex of the embryo is determined genetically at the time of fertilisation. However, it is not until the **7th week** that the gonads develop features of male or female morphology. **Primordial germ cells** migrate during the **5th week** of gestation from the yolk sac along the hindgut and its dorsal mesentery towards the mesenchyme of the posterior body wall. The mesonephros and coelomic epithelium proliferate to form a pair of **genital ridges**. During the **6th week**, cells of the genital ridge invade the mesenchyme to form **primitive sex cords**, consist-ing of cortical and medullary regions that will eventually invest the germ cells and support their development. At the same time, **paramesonephric ducts** develop lateral to the mesonephric ducts in a cranio-caudal direction. Primordial germ cells carry the XY sex chromosome if the embryo is genetically male. The **SRY gene** located on the Y chromosome encodes for **testis determin-ing factor**. This acts to stimulate proliferation of cells in the medulla and degeneration of cells in the cortical regions of the primitive sex cords. During the 7th week, the cells differentiate into **Sertoli cells** that become organised into testis cords and eventually to seminiferous tubules around the time of pubescence. These Sertoli cells secrete **Müllerian Inhibiting Substance** (MIS) that cause regression of the paramesonephric ducts between the 8th and 10th weeks, some of which remain as the Hydatid of Morgagni. Near the hilum, the testis cords break up into a net-work of thin strands that eventually become the rete testis. Some of these thin walled ducts con-nect to the mesonephric ducts from the medial aspect of the gonads. With further development, the testis cords become separated from the surface epithelium by the fibrous tunica albuginea. By the 10th week, **Leydig cells** develop from the mesenchymal cells of the genital ridge and secrete testosterone, initially under the influence of **placental chorionic gonadotropin** and later by the pituitary gonadotrophins. By the **12th week**, the mesonephric (Wolffian) duct is transformed into the vas deferens under the influence of testosterone. The cranial nephric duct also degenerates whilst the part adjacent to the presumptive testis becomes the epididymis. During the 7th week, the testes are located near the kidneys, held in position by the dorsal **cranial suspensory ligament** and the **ventral ligament**, which becomes the gubernaculum. During the 12th week, the testes descend to the inguinal canal and the suspensory ligament regresses. By the **28th week**, there is an outgrowth from the gubernaculum that passes through the external ring and enters the scrotum. It is hollowed out by a tongue of peritoneum (**processus vaginalis**), that allows the testes to descend into the scrotum by **33 weeks**. The peritoneal layer covering the testis becomes the visceral layer of the tunica vaginalis and the remainder of the peritoneal sac forms the parietal layer. The canal connecting the peritoneal cavity with the vaginal process becomes obliterated shortly before or after birth. The lack of testis determining factor in the female embryo causes the primitive sex cords to degenerate and the mesothelium of the genital ridge forms the secondary cortical sex cords. They invest the primordial germ cells to form ovarian follicles, which differentiate into oogonia and then primary oocytes that remain in this phase until puberty. The mesonephric ducts regress but the paramesonephric ducts develop into fallopian tubes, uterus and upper two-thirds of the vagina. The remainder of the inferior third of the vagina forms as a result of the caudal ends of the paramesonephric ducts, which come together and form a common channel (uterovaginal canal). It then fuses with the thickened tissue on the posterior urogenital sinus known as the sinovaginal bulb. The vaginal plate then develops at the inferior part of the canal, which then elongates and canalises between 12 and 20 weeks to form the inferior vaginal lumen.

Q7. Answer E

Each kidney measures 10–12 cm in length and weighs between 135 and 150 g. The right kidney is shorter and wider than the left and lies between the levels of the L1–L3 vertebrae from displacement by the liver. The left kidney lies up to 2 cm higher between T12 and L3. The **dromedary hump** is a bulge on the lateral contour of the kidney, more common on the left, caused by downward pressure from either the liver or spleen and is of no clinical significance. Each kidney is orientated in such a way that the upper poles are more medially and posteriorly located than the lower poles. Much of the surrounding relationship of each kidney is similar. The posterior upper third is covered by the diaphragm, the medial lower two-thirds lie against the psoas and the lateral contours are in contact with quadratus lumborum and the aponeurosis of transversus abdominis. Additionally, on the right, much of the medial aspect lies opposite the descending duodenum and the hepatic flexure of the colon cross over the anterior surface of the lower pole. On the left, the pancreatic tail reaches the upper pole and above this is the posterior gastric wall. The spleen is found on the outer upper aspect and is attached to the kidney by the splenorenal ligament. The splenic vessels lie adjacent to the hilum and the splenic flexure of the colon lies anterior to the lower pole. **Gerota's fascia** surrounds the kidney except inferiorly. Each kidney is divided into an outer thinner **cortex** and deeper thicker **medulla**. The medulla typically contains 7–9 renal pyramids whose apex (renal papillae) point towards the renal pelvis. Each papillae is cupped by a **minor calyx** and each drains via an infundibulum into two or three **major calyces**. These coalesce to form the renal pelvis that gives rise to the ureter. The cortex extends between the pyramids as **columns of Bertin** that contain the branching renal vasculature. Closely associated with these blood vessels are lymphatics that empty into larger trunks in the renal sinus before eventually reaching the lymph nodes closely associated with the renal veins. On the left, the lymphatic drainage is mainly to the lateral paraaortic nodes whilst on the right it is to the interaortocaval and paracaval nodes. The autonomic supply to the kidney is mainly concerned with vasomotor control; the sympathetic fibres originate from spinal nerves T8 to L1 and cause vasoconstriction whilst the vagal parasympathetic fibres cause vasodilation.

Q8. Answer E

The prostate develops during the 10th–12th week of gestation under influence of testosterone. The urogenital sinus gives off a prostatic bud comprised of solid epithelial cords, which canalise into solid prostatic ducts, and the epithelial cells become luminal and basal cells. The prostatic mesenchyme differentiates into smooth muscle cells to surround the ducts. There is a marked increase in the size of the prostate at puberty under the influence of testosterone and secretion of prostate specific antigen occurs. The gland is ovoid in shape, lies at the base of the bladder and weighs roughly 18 g in the normal adult. A fibrous capsule surrounds the gland composed of predominant **glandular tissue** (70%) and **fibromuscular stroma** (30%). It has an anterior, posterior and lateral surface with an inferior apex that lies on the urogenital diaphragm and a superior base. **The prostate is** further anatomically divided the gland into four zones based on the glandular elements.

1. **Peripheral** – Located posterior-laterally and forms the bulk of the gland. The ducts drain into the prostatic sinus. 75% of cancers arise from this zone.

2. **Central** – Cone-shaped zone that extends from around ejaculatory ducts to the base of the bladder.

3. **Transitional** – Surrounds the urethra and is separated from the other zones by a thin band of fibromuscular tissue. More commonly gives rise to *benign prostatic hyperplasia*.

4. **Anterior fibromuscular stroma** – Non-glandular segment extending from the bladder neck to the external urethral sphincter.

The rectum is posterior to the gland, separated by Denonvilliers' fascia and a loose layer of areolar tissue, the endopelvic fascia anterolaterally and the pubococcygeal muscles of levator ani laterally. Near the apex, the puboprostatic ligaments are on either side of the midline that extend from the prostate to the pubic bone. The base is continuous with the bladder neck where the detrusor muscle fibres merge with the capsule. The prostatic urethra is about 3 cm long and runs through the prostate from the bladder neck to become the membranous urethra. On the posterior wall, is a longitudinal ridge (urethral crest) that runs the length of the gland in between two grooves (prostatic sinus) into which the glandular elements open into the urethra. The crest widens distally to form the **verumontanum**. At its apex lies the slit-like prostatic utricle and represents a Müllerian remnant. The **ejaculatory ducts** open on either side of this. The main blood supply to the prostate is from the **inferior vesical artery**, which becomes the prostatic artery and divides into two main branches. The urethral arteries enter the prostate at the junction with the bladder and approach the bladder neck at the 1–11 (**Flock**) and 5–7 (**Badenoch**) o'clock positions. From here they run parallel to the urethra to supply the transition zone and periurethral glands. The capsular arteries supply the capsule and glandular tissues. The veins of the prostate drain into the dorsal vein complex lying just beneath the pubic symphysis; the deep dorsal vein leaves the penis under Buck's fascia and penetrates the urogenital diaphragm dividing into three major branches – the superficial branch and the right and left lateral plexus. The superficial branch pierces the endopelvic fascia and runs over the neck and anterior bladder surface to drain the anterior prostate, bladder and retropubic fat. The lateral branches pass down the sides of the prostate to join the vesical plexus, which subsequently drains into the internal iliac veins.

Q9. Answer B

The bladder has a dual function of storing and voiding urine with a capacity of 500 mL. Its shape changes with the amount of urine: a pyramidal shape when empty but ovoid when full. When empty, the apex faces anteriorly and lies just behind the pubic symphysis. It is the point of attachment for the **urachus**, a fibrous cord and remnant of the allantois, which suspends the bladder from the anterior abdominal wall by fusing with one of the obliterated umbilical arteries near the umbilicus. The base faces posteriorly, is triangular in shape and is in contact with a pair of seminal vesicles separated by the vas deferens. The inferior angle gives rise to the urethra. The bladder neck is 3–4 cm directly behind the pubic symphysis, and its position remains fixed during bladder distention. The superior surface is covered with peritoneum, which in women is further reflected over the uterus (vesicouterine pouch) and continues further back to cover the rectum (rectouterine pouch). On filling, the superior surface rises into the abdominal cavity, pushing the peritoneum away to come into direct contact with the posterior surface of the abdominal wall. The layers of bladder wall include an innermost transitional cell epithelium, made up to 6 cells thick overlying a basement membrane, the lamina propria and the outermost detrusor (smooth) muscle. The fibres of the detrusor are arranged into an inner longitudinal, circular and outer longitudinal fashion that forms the internal (proximal) sphincter. In men, the inner fibres are continuous with those of the urethra. The middle fibres form a ring around the bladder neck with the anterior fibromuscular stroma of the prostate. The outer fibres are abundant in the bladder base and they also form a loop around the bladder neck to provide continence. In females, the arrangement of the inner layer is similar but less is known about the arrangement of the middle and outer fibres. On approaching the bladder, the ureters become covered by a fibromuscular **Sheath of Waldeyer** before passing obliquely through the wall for about 2 cm and ending at the ureteral orifice. The intramural portion is narrow from compression by the detrusor muscle. This angle of entry and the surrounding detrusor muscle acts to prevent retrograde reflux of urine up the ureter. The two ureteric orifices form a triangular-shaped trigone with the apex at the bladder neck. The longitudinal muscle fibres of the ureter fan out over trigone and deep to this is the fibromuscular sheath of Waldeyer that inserts into the bladder neck. The urothelium is thinnest on the trigone. The fibres between the two orifices are thickened to form the interureteric ridge. The blood supply to the bladder is the superior and inferior vesical arteries. Venous drainage is to the vesical plexus, which drains into the internal iliac vein.

Q10. Answer E

The urethra extends from the bladder neck to the external meatus. It is longer in men (up to 20 cm) than in women (4 cm). In men, it is broadly divided into the anterior and posterior urethra. The latter is further subdivided into prostatic and membranous while anteriorly it is bulbar and pendulous. There are bends at the junctions between the membranous and bulbar and the bulbar and pendulous urethra. The membranous urethra is short and narrow as it passes through the urogenital diaphragm. It is surrounded by the striated external urethral sphincter whose inner smooth muscle is continuous with that of the proximal sphincter at the bladder neck. The outer muscle extends from the bladder neck and anterior prostate. The sphincter has a horseshoe configuration on cross section due to a broad anterior and a deficient posterior surface. Some of the fibres also attach to the perineal body causing the urethra to be pulled backwards when the sphincter contracts. The sphincter is also suspended from the pubic bones through attachments to the puboprostatic and suspensory ligament of the penis. Neural supply is from the somatic pudendal nerve and an autonomic branch from the sacral plexus. The anterior urethra is longer (15 cm), beginning at the level of the perineal membrane and transversing the whole length of the spongiosum to end at the narrow external meatus. It is dilated at the bulbar urethra and fossa navicularis in the glans. Mucus is secreted into the urethra by bulbourethral glands in the base of the external urethral sphincter and the glands of Littre in the submucosa. Proximally, the anterior urethra is lined by columnar epithelium but distally within the glans penis it is lined by stratified squamous epithelium. In contrast, the prostatic urethra is lined by transitional cell epithelium. The female urethra opens into the vestibule at the external meatus. On either side of the meatus are two ducts that drain mucus from the paraurethral (Skene) glands. It is surrounded by a striated external urethral sphincter. At the proximal and distal ends, the slow twitch muscle fibres completely surround the urethra whilst the fibres in the middle do not meet posteriorly and instead attach to the vagina. The urethra is pulled against the vagina when the sphincter contracts. The urethra is suspended beneath the pubic bone by the suspensory ligament of clitoris and the pubourethral ligament. It is lined proximally by transitional cell epithelium, which becomes stratified squamous epithelium distally. Somatic nerve innervation is similar to that in the male.

EMQs – ANSWERS

Q11. Answers

1F, 2A, 3B, 4E, 5C, 6D, 7I, 8J, 9K, 10I

The female reproductive tract is made up of the uterus, a pair of ovaries and fallopian tubes, and the vagina. The uterus measures roughly 8 × 6 cm and lies in front of the rectum and over the dome of the bladder. It consists of the upper fundus, middle body and lower cervix. It is anchored by the **round ligament of uterus,** which originates at the uterine horns, leaves the pelvis at the deep inguinal ring, passes through the inguinal canal and continues on to the labia majora where its fibres attach to the mons pubis. Each fallopian tube extends laterally from the side of the uterus at the junction between the fundus and body. There are four anatomical parts:

- **Infundibulum** – 'Funnel shaped' lateral end, which opens into the peritoneal cavity. Fimbriae surround the mouth of the tube to collect ova from the ovary.
- **Ampulla** – Site of fertilisation.
- **Isthmus** – Involved with the transport of gametes in both directions.
- **Uterine** – Within the wall of the uterus.

The fallopian tubes protrude upwards and lift the peritoneum into a fold known as the **broad ligament** that connects the sides of the uterus to the pelvic walls and floor. The **cardinal (Mackenrodt's) ligament** is located in the base of the broad ligament and attaches the cervix to the lateral pelvic wall at the ischial spine and carries the uterine vessels. Each ovary sits in a fossa on the lateral wall of the pelvis surrounded by the external iliac vessels above, the internal iliac vessels and ureter behind and the obturator nerve in the floor. Each ovary is secured to a different structure by several ligaments;

- **Mesovarium ligament** – To the back of the broad ligament.
- **Round ligament of ovary** – To the side of the uterus by passing through the broad ligament.
- **Suspensory ligament** – To the pelvic side wall and carries the ovarian artery.

The vagina measures approximately 8 cm in length and is a muscular tube connecting the vulva to the uterus. The cervix pierces the upper anterior wall of the vagina, which lies above the pelvic floor. The space surrounding the cervix is divided into the anterior, posterior, right and left lateral fornices. The vagina is lined by non-keratinised squamous epithelium and surrounded by smooth muscle. The surrounding anatomical relationships include the lateral levator ani muscles, and posteriorly the Pouch of Douglas at the upper third, ampulla of the rectum in the middle third and the anal canal at the lower third. The vagina and rectum are separated by a septum, deep to which is the rectovaginal space. The bladder base rests on the vaginal wall immediately in front of the cervix and is held in place by strong muscle fibres.

The blood supply to the female organs mainly originates from branches of the internal iliac artery; the **vaginal artery** provides the main supply to the vagina whilst the **uterine artery**, which runs in front of the ureter and in the cardinal ligament, supplies the proximal vagina, uterus and part of the fallopian tubes. The ovarian arteries usually arise from the aorta below the renal arteries at the level of L1, but in a small number may originate from the renal artery. It descends over the psoas and in the pelvis runs in the suspensory ligament to anastomose with the ovarian branch of the uterine artery supplying the ovary.

Q12. Answers

1B, 2A, 3C, 4H, 5E, 6I, 7F, 8D, 9G, 10J, 11K

The embryological development of the urinary system passes through three main stages: the **pronephros, mesonephros** and **metanephros**. The process begins with the **intermediate mesoderm**, a ridge-like structure located on either side of the midline notochord and neural tube along the posterior abdominal cavity. The cervical and upper thoracic portions of this ridge are segmented but unsegmented in the lower thoracic, lumbar and sacral regions and known as the **nephrogenic cord**. Caudally, the nephrogenic cord, and later the mesonephric ducts, drain into an endoderm lined yolk sac known as the **cloaca**. This develops from the cloacal membrane during the 4th week but, by the 6th week, its cavity has divided into the anterior **urogenital sinus**, which becomes the bladder and urethra, and the posterior **anorectal canal**. The **pronephros** is a temporary non-functioning unit that develops during week 3 at the cranial end of the intermediate mesoderm and regresses by the end of the 4th week, that consists of 6–10 pairs of pronephric tubules that mature, starting at the cranial end and then regress as more caudal tubules develop. The **mesonephros** then forms from the 4th week in the middle part of the intermediate mesoderm that acts as the excretory organ for the embryo. Thereafter, it degenerates leaving behind parts of the duct system to form the male reproductive organs. Whilst the mesonephros is developing, a pair of **mesonephric (Wolffian) duct** form on either side that fuse caudally with the cloaca. Between 40 and 42 pairs of (mesonephric) tubules arise from the mesonephros that elongate and join laterally with the mesonephric ducts. The medial end of the tubule is cup-shaped and accepts a sphere of capillaries to form a **Bowman's capsule**. At the start of the 5th week, the tubules begin to degenerate in a cranial to caudal direction, but some remain to become the efferent ductules of the testes. The epididymis, vas deferens, seminal vesicles and ejaculatory ducts all develop from persistence of the mesonephric ducts. At the end of the 5th week, the **metanephros** begins its development, eventually differentiating into the kidney. A pair of **paramesonephric (Müllerian) ducts** develop lateral to the mesonephric ducts. They extend from the urogenital sinus to the level of the 3rd thoracic segment where the cranial ends open into the coelomic cavity. In males, these ducts eventually degenerate, however, in females they become the fallopian tubes, uterus, cervix and upper two-thirds of the vagina. The **ureteric bud** becomes the ureter, renal pelvis, calyces and collecting ducts. It arises from the distal end of the mesonephric duct and penetrates the adjacent metanephric tissue. Its tip (ampulla) divides dichotomously to give rise to the metanephric tissue that will become the glomeruli and nephrons. The first division of the ampulla defines the primitive renal pelvis and the future major calyces. The buds then continue to divide towards the periphery until 12 or more generations of collecting tubules have been formed. The first five generations of tubules dilate and develop into the pelvis and calyces. Successive generations elongate to become the renal pyramids. At the periphery, tubular formation continues until the end of the 5th month. The metanephric mesenchyme, in contact with the tips of the collecting tubule, condense and then elongate. One end forms Bowman's capsule whilst the other forms an open connection with the collecting tubule. Although urine production starts at week 10, nephron formation continues throughout the developing kidney until the 32nd to 34th week. The developing kidneys migrate upwards from the 6th week to reach the lumbar region below the adrenals by week nine. Arteries arise from the aorta and then regress as they supply the kidneys, which migrate superiorly to their destination where the definitive renal arteries will develop.

Q13. Answers

1E, 2H, 3A, 4B, 5G, 6F, 7J, 8I, 9D, 10C

The bony pelvis protects the distal ends of the gastrointestinal and urinary systems, and the internal reproductive organs. The anterior and lateral walls are made up of two hip bones that meet anteriorly at the symphysis pubis and posteriorly with the sacrum at the sacroiliac joints. The sacrum and coccyx form the back wall. The pelvis is often divided into the true and false pelvis. The former lies below the pelvic brim, and consists of an inlet, outlet and cavity. The inlet is surrounded by the sacral promontory posteriorly, iliopectineal lines laterally and the pubic symphysis anteriorly. In contrast, the outlet is bounded by the coccyx behind, ischial tuberosities laterally and the pubic arch anteriorly. The false pelvis lies above the pelvic brim to form part of the lower abdominal cavity. The boundaries include the lumbar vertebrae behind, iliac fossa and iliacus laterally, and the abdominal wall anteriorly. The greater and lesser sciatic notches lie behind the acetabulum and are separated by the ischial spines. The greater and lesser sciatic foramina are formed by two muscles; sacrotuberous extends from the sacrum, coccyx and posterior inferior iliac spine to the ischial tuberosity, whilst sacrospinous extends from the sacrum and coccyx to the ischial spine. The obturator foramen is surrounded by the pubic bone above and ischium below and is filled by a fibrous sheet through which the obturator nerve and vessels pass as they enter the thigh. Attached to this sheet is the obturator internus muscle that gives rise to a tendon that leaves the pelvis through the lesser sciatic foramen and attaches to the greater trochanter of the femur. The pelvic floor supports the pelvic organs and separates them from the perineum. Anteriorly, the floor is incomplete allowing the urethra to pass through and in females the vagina (urogenital hiatus). It is made up of two main muscle groups: levator ani made up of several structures and also the smaller coccygeus muscle. Levator ani originates from the back of the pubic bone, ischial spine and the thickened fascia of obturator internus and is supplied by the perineal branches of the 4th sacral and pudendal nerves. The anterior levator prostate, or sphincter vaginae, which attach to the perineal body either form a sling around and support the prostate, or surround the vagina, respectively. Puborectalis and pubococcygeus lie behind and form a sling that serves as a sphincter around the junction of the rectum and anal canal. Posteriorly is iliococcygeus, which attaches to the anococcygeal body in a similar way to pubococcygeus. Coccygeus is the most posterior muscle that is supplied by the 4th and 5th sacral nerves and arises from the ischial spine extending to the sacrum and coccyx. The pelvic fascia is made of collagen, elastic tissue and smooth muscle. It is continuous above with the fascia of the abdominal wall and below with the fascia of the perineum. The parietal layer lines the walls of the pelvis and its muscles. Anteriorly, at the urogenital hiatus, the fascia becomes continuous with that of the perineum. The visceral layer covers and supports the pelvic organs. In some areas it is thickened to form ligaments that support organs. The puboprostatic ligament attaches at the junction of the prostate and external sphincter to the back of the pubic bone. In females, the equivalent is the pubourethral ligament, which attaches to the proximal third of the urethra. Another ligament is the arcus tendineus fascia pelvis, which extends from the puboprostatic/pubourethral ligament to the ischial spine and has the lateral branches of the dorsal vein complex beneath it. The urogenital diaphragm supports the urethral sphincter above and is a point of attachment for the external genitalia below. It extends from the pubic symphysis to the ischial tuberosities and covers the urogenital hiatus from below. At its centre lies the triangular-shaped perineal membrane. Posteriorly, the transverse perineal muscles run along its free edge. The perineal body lies just behind the diaphragm and serves as a point of attachment for almost all pelvic muscles and fascia and is therefore important in providing pelvic support. The perineum is 'rhomboid shaped' when viewed from below. The pubic symphysis lies anteriorly, with the coccyx at the back and the ischial tuberosities laterally to make up its four corners. The perineum is also divided into an anterior urogenital triangle and a posterior anal triangle by an imaginary line connecting both ischial tuberosities. The boundaries of the urogenital triangle are the pubic arch anteriorly and the ischial tuberosities laterally. Camper's fascia lies below the skin covering the perineum and overlies the deeper Colles' fascia. The urogenital diaphragm bridges the urogenital triangle. The superficial perineal pouch is a space between the urogenital diaphragm and Colles' fascia where the root of the penis originates. The space can also communicate with another potential space lying in between the fascia and muscles of the anterior abdominal wall. The blood supply to the perineum includes the perineal branch of the internal pudendal artery with branches of the pudendal nerve providing sensory innervation to the area.

Q14. Answers

1I, 2G, 3B, 4J, 5A, 6H, 7D, 8C, 9E, 10F

The autonomic nervous system provides sympathetic and parasympathetic supply to organs, blood vessels, glands and smooth muscle. The somatic system innervates skin, skeletal muscles and joints. Parasympathetic fibres arise from cranial and sacral spinal nerves, whilst sympathetic fibres for the thoracolumbar region originate from spinal nerves T1 to L3. The two sympathetic chains lie anteriorly on either side of the vertebral column to which the preganglionic fibres synapse. These fibres then continue via splanchnic nerves to the coeliac or superior and inferior plexuses associated with the aorta to synapse with postganglionic fibres that supply the target organ. Preganglionic fibres also directly supply the adrenal gland. The coeliac plexus is closely associated with the coeliac trunk and is where a significant proportion of the autonomic supply to the kidneys, adrenals, renal pelvis and ureters pass through. The superior hypogastric plexus lies below this near the aortic bifurcation and connects with the inferior hypogastric plexus below. Any disruption here during retroperitoneal lymph node dissection can result in retrograde ejaculation. The somatic lumbosacral plexus is formed from spinal nerves L1 to S3 and provides innervation to the abdomen and lower extremities. The major nerves of the plexus are described in the following table.

Nerve	Origins	Course	Function
Iliohypogastric	Superior branch of the anterior ramus of L1	Emerges from the upper psoas and crosses in front of quadratus lumborum to the iliac crest. It pierces transversus abdominis, and divides into lateral and anterior cutaneous branches.	**Sensory:** Skin of the gluteal and pubic region. **Motor:** Internal oblique and transversus abdominis.
Ilioinguinal	Inferior branch of the anterior ramus of L1	Similar route to the iliohypogastric nerve but below it. Pierces the internal oblique muscle and then accompanies the spermatic cord through the superficial inguinal ring travels partway through the inguinal canal.	**Sensory:** *Male:* Skin over the root of the penis and anterior scrotum. *Female:* Skin covering the mons pubis and labia majora. **Motor:** Internal oblique and transversus abdominis.
Genitofemoral	Anterior rami of L1–L2	Emerges from the anterior surface of psoas and divides into femoral and genital branches.	**Femoral branch:** Sensation to the skin overlying the femoral triangle. **Genital branch:** *Male:* Travels with the spermatic cord in the inguinal canal and supplies the cremaster and dartos muscles (cremasteric reflex) and the scrotal skin. *Female:* Sensation to the skin of the mons pubis and labia majora.
Lateral cutaneous nerve of the thigh	Anterior rami of L2–L3	Emerges from the lateral psoas and crosses the iliacus muscle, passing under the inguinal ligament and over the sartorius muscle into the thigh.	**Sensory:** Skin of the anterior and lateral aspect of the thigh.

(*Continued*)

Nerve	Origins	Course	Function
Obturator	Anterior rami of L2–L4	Descends through the psoas and emerges from its medial border. It then passes behind the common iliac arteries, runs along the lateral wall of the pelvis and passes through the obturator foramen to enter the thigh through the obturator canal to split into anterior & posterior branches.	**Sensory:** Skin of the medial aspect of the thigh. **Motor:** Adductor muscles of lower extremity.
Femoral	Anterior rami of L2–L4	Descends through the psoas and emerges from its lateral lower border. It then passes over the iliacus muscle and under the inguinal ligament to enter the thigh.	**Sensory:** Skin of the anterior thigh and medial leg. **Motor:** Supplies pectineus, sartorius and quadriceps femoris.

Q15. Answers

1D, 2G, 3A, 4H, 5B, 6F, 7J, 8C, 9E, 10I

The abdominal aorta lies in the retroperitoneum on the anterior surface of the vertebral bodies. It is a continuation of the thoracic aorta, where it passes through the aortic hiatus between the diaphragmatic crura at the level of T12. It continues down to the level of L4, where it bifurcates into the paired common iliac arteries. Moving down the aorta in the caudal direction, **inferior phrenic arteries** are the first branches of the abdominal aorta and supply the diaphragm and adrenal glands. The next branch to arise is the **coeliac trunk**, which gives rise to the common hepatic, left gastric and splenic arteries. The paired **adrenal arteries** are the next to branch. Below this is the **superior mesenteric artery** that supplies the small bowel and part of the large bowel. The **renal arteries** are the next to branch from the aorta at the level of L2. The paired **testicular (or ovarian in women) arteries** originate just below the renal arteries. They cross over the ureter as they run towards the deep inguinal ring to leave the abdomen. The ovarian artery does not enter the inguinal canal but passes over the iliac vessels and proceeds to the ovary via the suspensory ligament. Both the testes and ovaries have a collateral blood supply, which means they can be sacrificed during surgery. The **inferior mesenteric artery** supplies the remainder of the large bowel and is the next branch of the aorta. Due to its collateral circulation, it can be ligated without any detrimental effects on the bowel. The final branch, just before the aortic bifurcation, is the **middle sacral artery**, which supplies the anterior sacrum and rectum. Pairs of lumbar arteries (typically four) are given off along the lateral aspect of the aorta to supply the spinal cord and posterior body wall. The **common iliac arteries** run laterally and bifurcate anterior to the sacroiliac joint into the **internal and external iliac arteries**. The external iliac arteries run along the medial border of the psoas and become the femoral arteries below the level of the inguinal ligament just before giving rise to the **deep circumflex iliac and inferior epigastric arteries**. The inferior epigastric artery runs upwards, medial to the deep inguinal ring, to supply the rectus abdominis and skin of the anterior abdominal wall. An **accessory obturator artery** is found in a quarter of subjects and arises from the inferior epigastric artery that runs medially to the femoral vein to reach the obturator canal. The internal iliac artery divides into an anterior and posterior trunk and their branches are listed in the table below.

Anterior Trunk	
Umbilical	The proximal portion gives rise to the **superior vesical** artery, which supplies the upper portion of the bladder, seminal vesicles and vas deferens.
Inferior vesical	Supplies the ureter, bladder base, prostate and seminal vesicles (vagina in females).
Middle rectal	Supplies the prostate and seminal vesicles. Joins the superior and inferior rectal arteries to supply the rectum.
Internal pudendal	Leaves the pelvis through the greater sciatic foramen, passes behind sacrospinous ligament and enters the pelvis again through the lesser sciatic foramen to reach the perineum. It passes forward in the pudendal canal with the pudendal nerve to supply the anal canal and skin/muscles of the perineum.
Inferior gluteal	Exits the pelvis through the greater sciatic foramen to supply the gluteal and thigh muscles.
Uterine	Passes superiorly and anteriorly to the ureter and runs up the lateral wall of the uterus in the broad ligament and then follows the fallopian tube laterally where it joins the ovarian artery.
Vaginal	Supplies the vagina.
Obturator	Runs along the lateral wall of the pelvis with the obturator nerve and leaves the pelvis through the obturator canal to supply the adductors of the thigh.
Posterior Trunk	
Superior gluteal	Leaves the pelvis through the greater sciatic foramen to supply the gluteal muscles.
Iliolumbar	Supplies iliacus, psoas, quadratus lumborum and cauda equina anastomosing with the last lumbar artery.
Lateral sacral	Runs down in front of the sacral plexus joining the middle sacral artery to supply neighbouring structures.

The common iliac veins join at the level of L5 posteriorly and to the right of the aortic bifurcation. The first tributary of the inferior vena cava (IVC) is the middle sacral vein then the gonadal, renal, adrenal and hepatic veins moving cranially. The IVC receives multiple lumbar veins along its posterior aspect. The right gonadal, adrenal and inferior phrenic veins drain into the IVC whereas on the left side, these drain into the left renal vein.

CHAPTER 2: RENAL PATHOPHYSIOLOGY

Herman S. Fernando, Mohamed Yehia Abdallah and Iqbal S. Shergill

MCQs

Q1. Which of the following is CORRECT regarding the nephron?

A. The glomerulus is about 20 μm in diameter and is formed by the invagination of a tuft of capillaries into the dilated, open end of the nephron (Bowman's capsule).

B. Functionally, the glomerular basement membrane permits the free passage of neutral substances upto 4 nm in diameter and totally excludes those with diameters greater than 8 nm.

C. In the distal convoluted tubule, while the predominant principle cells (P) are involved in acid secretion and HCO_3^- transport, the intercalated cells (I) are associated with Na^+ reabsorption and vasopressin-stimulated water reabsorption.

D. The renin-secreting juxtaglomerular cells are situated in that part of the thick ascending limb of the loop of Henle, which traverses close to the afferent arteriole from which the tubule arose.

E. In a resting adult, the kidneys receive about 450 mL of blood per minute.

Q2. Which of the following is CORRECT regarding GFR?

A. The best estimate of GFR can be obtained by measuring the rate of clearance of a given substance from the plasma, and inulin clearance is felt to be the best measure of GFR.

B. 24-hour creatinine clearance overestimates true GFR by 5%, and thus, as GFR declines, tubular secretion increases in response to increasing creatinine levels may contribute upto 10%–15% of all creatinine levels at GFR levels of 40–80 mL/min. At best, then, the CrCL should be considered the 'upper limit' of the true GFR.

C. Cockcroft-Gault measures creatinine clearance by the formula:
CrCl = {[(140 − age) × (Lean Body Weight in kg)]/[Serum Creatinine (mg/dL) × 72]} × 1.05 (women).

D. The simplest estimate of GFR is the four-variable equation (PCr, weight, sex and ethnicity), which estimates GFR using the formula: eGFR (mL/min/1.73 m) = 186 × (Serum Creatinine [mg/dL])$^{-1.154}$ × (weight in kg)$^{-0.203}$ × (0.742 if female) × (1.210 if African American).

E. MDRD, which is used to calculate the eGFR is not validated for use in children, whilst CG formula overestimates CrCl in children due to reabsorption.

Q3. Which of the following is TRUE regarding bone mineralisation?

A. The actions of Vitamin D are exerted largely through the liver.

B. Vitamin D3 requires two hydroxylations, first in liver and second in the kidney.

C. During periods of hypercalcemia, PTH synthesis and secretion are increased while degradation is decreased.

D. The renal effects of PTH are to increase active calcium reabsorption at the level of the proximal tubule and decrease phosphate reabsorption mainly in the distal tubule.

E. PTH stimulates calcitriol production by decreasing 1α-hydroxylase levels.

Q4. **Which of the following is TRUE in unilateral ureteric obstruction (UUO)?**

A. Renal blood flow (RBF) increases during the first 1 1/2 to 4 hours along with an increase in the ureteric pressure.

B. In a second phase lasting between 3 and 5 hours, these pressure parameters remain elevated but RBF begins to rapidly decline.

C. A third phase beginning about 5 hours after obstruction is associated with a further drop in RBF and a gradual but small rise in collecting system pressure.

D. Infusion of Captopril, an ACE inhibitor attenuates the declines in RBF and GFR in UUO.

E. Administration of endothelin antagonists limits the reduction of RBF but increases GFR in rats during and after release of UUO.

Q5. **Regarding ureteric obstruction, which is CORRECT?**

A. In UUO, blocking nitric oxide (NO) release contributes to renal vasoconstriction.

B. In UUO, Thromboxane A2 (TXA2) administration causes reduction of GFR and rise in RBF.

C. In bilateral ureteric obstruction (BUO), there occurs a prolonged increase in RBF that lasts for nearly 4–5 hours.

D. In BUO, blood flows from inner to outer cortex.

E. Compared to UOO, in BUO accumulation of substances like atrial natriuretic peptide (ANP) leads to preglomerular vasodilation and postglomerular vasoconstriction.

Q6. **Regarding post-obstructive diuresis, which of the following is FALSE?**

A. Although this occurs mainly after relief of BUO or obstruction of a solitary kidney, it can rarely occur when there is a normal contralateral kidney.

B. The normal physiologic diuretic response is due to the volume expansion and solute accumulation occurring during obstruction.

C. A pathological postobstructive diuresis, characterised by inappropriate renal handling of water or solutes occurs due to a derangement of the medullary solute gradient and downregulation of sodium transporters with subsequent impaired sodium reabsorption in the distal convoluted tubule.

D. There is no role for gradual bladder decompression, because this has not been demonstrated to limit hematuria or reduce the risk of postobstructive diuresis.

E. Pathologic postobstructive diuresis is also marked by poor responsiveness of the collecting duct to antidiuretic hormone (ADH).

Q7. **Regarding retroperitoneal fibrosis (RPF), which of the following is FALSE?**

A. One possible pathogenesis could be the development of vasculitis in the adventitial vessels of the aorta and periaortic small vessels.

B. Inflammatory bowel disease (IBD) is reported to be a cause of RPF.

C. The classic radiologic findings include medial deviation of extrinsically compressed ureters with hydronephrosis.

D. CT typically reveals a well demarcated retroperitoneal mass, isodense to muscle on unenhanced studies.

E. Tamoxifen, a steroidal anti-oestrogen, has also been used for primary treatment at a dose of 20 mg per day with a reported response rate of 80%.

Q8. **Which of the following is TRUE in hydronephrosis of pregnancy?**

A. The reported occurrence varies between 5% and 15%.

B. The right kidney becomes hydronephrotic two to three times more commonly than the left.

C. Approximately one half of patients have persistent hydronephrosis during the first postpartum week, but it resolves within 2 weeks of delivery in the majority.

D. The use of MRI is advocated in the first trimester of pregnancy but gadolinium contrast should be avoided because it crosses the placental barrier.

E. The majority of patients with symptomatic hydronephrosis of pregnancy can be managed with placement of ureteral stents or nephrostomy (especially if associated with pyonephrosis).

Q9. **Which of the following is FALSE regarding biochemical pathology of urine in patients with kidney stones?**

A. A solution containing ions or molecules of a sparingly soluble salt is described by the *concentration product*, which is a mathematic expression of the product of the concentrations of the pure chemical components (ions or molecules) of the salt.

B. The concentration product, the point at which the dissolved and crystalline components are in equilibrium for a specific set of conditions, at the point of saturation is called the *stability product*, Ksp.

C. The Ksp value and the formation product (Kf) differentiate the three major states of saturation in urine: undersaturated, metastable, and unstable.

D. The concentration product at the point where the crystals can no longer be held in solution is called the *formation product*, Kf.

E. Inhibitors can generally prevent the process of crystal growth or aggregation above the *formation product*, Kf.

Q10. **Which of the following is TRUE regarding biochemical pathology of urine?**

A. Tamm-Horsfall protein is secreted by renal epithelial cells in the loop of Henle and the proximal convoluted tubule as a membrane-anchored protein.

B. Nephrocalcin is an acidic glycoprotein containing predominantly acidic amino acids that is synthesised in the thick ascending limb and distal tubule.

C. Uropontin is an acidic phosphorylated glycoprotein expressed in bone matrix and renal epithelial cells of the ascending limb of the loop of Henle and the distal tubule.

D. Polyanions including glycosaminoglycans, acid mucopolysaccharides and RNA have been shown to inhibit crystal growth but not nucleation.

E. Among the glycosaminoglycans, heparan sulfate interacts most strongly with calcium phosphate crystals.

Q11. **Which of the following is FALSE regarding biochemical pathology of urine?**

A. Tamm-Horsfall is the most abundant protein found in the urine and a potent inhibitor of calcium oxalate monohydrate crystal growth and aggregation.

B. Nephrocalcin strongly inhibits the growth of calcium oxalate monohydrate crystals.

C. Osteopontin has been shown to inhibit nucleation, growth and aggregation of calcium oxalate crystals.

D. The inhibitory activity of magnesium is derived from its complexation with oxalate.

E. Heparan sulfate interacts most strongly with calcium oxalate monohydrate crystals.

Q12. **Which of the following is FALSE regarding renal tubular acidosis (RTA)?**

A. In Type I RTA, there is failure of H^+ secretion in the distal nephron.

B. Type I RTA is associated with hyperchloremic metabolic acidosis with a high urinary pH and persistently low HCO_3.

C. Type I patients do not have a tendency to develop stones.

D. Type I RTA may be associated with chronic ureteric obstruction, autoimmune thyroiditis and toxic nephropathy.

E. The medical treatment of RTA aims to alkalinise the urine with sodium bicarbonate.

Q13. **Which of the following agents do NOT have a vasoconstrictor effect on renal artery?**

A. Angiotensin II
B. Vasopressin
C. Endothelin
D. Atrial natriuretic peptide
E. Serotonin/bradykinin

Q14. Which of the following factors do NOT stimulate the release of ADH?
A. Stress
B. Hyperosmolality
C. Hypervolemia
D. Hypoglycemia
E. Pregnancy

Q15. The following are common causes of hyperkalemia EXCEPT for:
A. Renal failure
B. Drugs including digoxin, angiotensin-converting enzyme [ACE] inhibitors
C. Chronic acidosis
D. TUR syndrome
E. Hypoaldosteronism

Q16. The following medications are associated with retroperitoneal fibrosis EXCEPT for:
A. Methysergide
B. Hydralazine
C. Alpha-blockers
D. Haloperidol
E. Phenacetin

Q17. The following drugs cause acute interstitial nephritis EXCEPT for:
A. Nonsteroidal anti-inflammatory drugs
B. Cephalosporins
C. Rifampin
D. Ciprofloxacin
E. Bicalutamide

EMQs

Q18–26. Sodium levels in the human body
   A. Low total body sodium
   B. High total body sodium
   C. Normal total body sodium
For each of the following conditions below, select the most appropriate option from the list above. Each option may be used once, more than once or not at all.

Q18. Loop diuretics

Q19. Cushing syndrome

Q20. Osmotic diuretic

Q21. Hypertonic dialysis

Q22. Nephrogenic diabetes insipidus

Q23. Central diabetes insipidus

Q24. GI fistula

Q25. Diarrhoea

Q26. Hyperaldosteronism

Q27–33. Drugs used in renal transplant patients
   A. Inhibits purine synthesis
   B. Inhibits cell cycle progression
   C. Inhibits calcineurin
   D. Blocks IL-2 receptor

For each of the following drugs used in renal transplantation below, select the most appropriate mode of action from the list above. Each option may be used once, more than once or not at all.

Q27. Mycophenolate mofetil

Q28. Sirolimus

Q29. Cyclosporin

Q30. Basiliximab

Q31. Daclizumab

Q32. Tacrolimus

Q33. Azathioprine

Q34–40. Medical therapy in renal cancer
   A. Multikinase inhibitor
   B. Tyrosine kinase inhibitor
   C. Monoclonal antibody to VEGF
   D. Angiogenesis inhibitor
   E. EGF family receptor blocker
   F. Oral mTOR inhibitor
For each of the following therapies used for renal cancer below, select the most appropriate mode of action from the list above. Each option may be used once, more than once or not at all.

Q34. Sorafenib

Q35. Bevacizumab

Q36. Lapatinib

Q37. Pazopanib

Q38. Everolimus

Q39. Sunitinib

Q40. Temsirolimus

Q41–49. Metabolic acidosis and anion gap
   A. Normal anion gap
   B. Increased anion gap

For each of the following descriptions below, select the most appropriate option from the list above. Each option may be used once, more than once or not at all.

Q41. Hyperalimentation therapy

Q42. Salicylate poisoning

Q43. Diabetic ketoacidosis

Q44. Diarrhoea

Q45. Proximal renal tubular acidosis

Q46. Distal renal tubular acidosis

Q47. Chronic renal failure

Q48. Cholestyramine therapy

Q49. Lactic acidosis

Q50–56. Chemotherapeutic agents in urologic oncology
   A. Antimetabolite
   B. Antimitotic
   C. Antibiotic
   D. Alkylating agent

For each of the following drugs used in uro-oncology below, select the most appropriate mode of action from the list above. Each option may be used once, more than once or not at all.

Q50. Cisplatin

Q51. Vincristine

Q52. Taxane

Q53. Methotrexate

Q54. 5-Fluorouracil

Q55. Bleomycin

Q56. Cyclophosphamide

Q57–62. Inherited urological conditions and chromosome associations
   A. Chromosome 9
   B. Chromosome 2
   C. Chromosome 14
   D. Chromosome 6
   E. Chromosome 19
   F. Chromosome 4
   G. Chromosome 1
   H. Chromosome 17

For each of the following inherited urological conditions below, select the most appropriate chromosome from the list above. Each option may be used once, more than once or not at all.

Q57. Papillary renal cell cancer type 2, Chromosome 1

Q58. 5 alpha reductase deficiency, Chromosome 2

Q59. Cystinuria, Chromosome 2

Q60. Autosomal dominant polycystic kidney disease, Chromosomes 4 and 16

Q61. Autosomal recessive polycystic kidney disease, Chromosome 6

Q62. Tuberous sclerosis, Chromosome 9

Q63–68. Half-life of commonly used urological drugs
   A. 5 days
   B. 5 seconds
   C. 2 weeks
   D. 4 hours
   E. 6 hours
   F. 1 month
   G. 3 months

For each of the following drugs listed below, select the most appropriate answer from the list above. Each option may be used once, more than once or not at all.

Q63. Goserelin

Q64. Sildenafil

Q65. Bicalutamide

Q66. AFP

Q67. Tc99m

Q68. Nitric oxide

MCQs – ANSWERS

Q1. Answer B

The glomerulus, which is about 200 μm in diameter, is formed by the invagination of a tuft of capillaries into the dilated, blind end of the nephron. In the distal convoluted tubule, while the predominant principle cells (P) are involved in Na^+ reabsorption and vasopressin-stimulated water reabsorption, the intercalated cells (I) are associated with acid secretion and HCO_3^- transport. It is the wall of the afferent arteriole that contains renin-secreting juxtaglomerular cells. At this point the wall of the tubular epithelium is modified histologically to become the macula densa. The juxtaglomerular cells, the macula densa and the lacis cells near them are collectively known as juxtaglomerular apparatus. The kidney receives 25% of cardiac output.

Q2. Answer A

The 24-hour creatinine clearance (CrCl) overestimates true GFR by 10%–20% and thus as GFR declines, tubular secretion increases in response to increasing creatinine levels may contribute upto 35% of all creatinine levels at GFR levels of 40–80 mL/min. At best, then, the CrCL should be considered the 'upper limit' of the true GFR. Cockcroft-Gault measures creatinine clearance by the formula – CrCl = {[(140-age) × (Lean Body Weight in kg)]/[Serum Creatinine (mg/dL) × 72]} × 0.85 (women). It underestimates CrCL in children due to reabsorption. Moreover, the calculation is dependent on accurate collection of the specimen, which can be incomplete. The MDRD formula to estimate GFR is eGFR (in mL/min/1.73 m) = 186 × (Serum Creatinine $[mg/dL])^{-1.154}$ × $(age)^{-0.203}$ × (0.742 if female) × (1.210 if African American). However, this formula is not validated for use in children, whilst Cockcroft-Gault formula overestimates CrCl in children due to reabsorption.

Q3. Answer B

Normal regulation of bone mineralisation occurs through maintenance of serum calcium and phosphorus levels and is achieved through the actions of vitamin D and parathyroid hormone (PTH). The actions of both hormones are exerted largely through the kidney. Vitamin D3, which has minimal biological activity, requires two hydroxylations – first occurs in the liver and the second within the tubular cell, through the action of 25-hydroxylase to form 25-hydroxycholecalciferol (calcidiol). The calcidiol is then transported to the kidney, where it is filtered and reabsorbed by renal tubular cells. These cells contain both 1α-hydroxylase and 24α-hydroxylase, and produce either the active 1,25-dihydroxycholecalciferol (calcitriol) or the inactive 24,25-dihydroxycholecalciferol. Parathormone increases the active calcium reabsorption at the level of the distal tubule. Secondly, it decreases phosphate reabsorption in the proximal convoluted tubule (and the distal tubule, to a lesser degree) and thirdly, it stimulates calcitriol production by increasing 1α-hydoxylase levels and decreasing 24α-hydroxylase levels.

Q4. Answer D

In UUO, RBF increases during the first 0–90 minutes and is accompanied by a high collecting system pressure because of the obstruction. In the second phase lasting up to 5 hours, both RBF and collecting system pressure remain elevated but RBF begins to gradually decline. A third phase beginning about 5 hours after obstruction is characterised by a further decline in RBF, now paralleled by a decrease in collecting system pressure.

Infusion of the angiotensin-converting enzyme (ACE) inhibitor Captopril attenuates the declines in RBF and GFR in UUO, suggesting that angiotensin II is an important mediator of the preglomerular vasoconstriction in the second and third phases of UUO. Endothelin antagonists limit the reduction of RBF and GFR in rats during and after release of UUO.

Q5. Answer E

In UUO, both PGE2 and NO contribute to the net renal vasodilation that occurs early following UUO. Studies have shown that the increase in PGE2 and the vasodilation of the obstructed kidney is blocked by indomethacin, a prostaglandin synthesis inhibitor. TXA2 is an influential postobstructive vasoconstrictor that contributes to the continued reduction in GFR and RBF. Administration of TXA2 synthesis inhibitors to the obstructed kidney limits the reduction in RBF and GFR.

In contrast to the early robust renal vasodilation with UUO, there is a modest increase in RBF with BUO that lasts approximately 90 minutes, followed by a prolonged and profound decrease in RBF that is greater than found with UUO. The shift seen with UUO of blood flow from outer to inner cortex is the opposite of that with BUO.

This difference between BUO and UUO could be due to an accumulation of vasoactive substances like ANP in BUO and this could contribute to preglomerular vasodilation and postglomerular vasoconstriction. Such substances do not accumulate in UUO because they would be excreted by the contralateral kidney.

Q6. Answer C

POD in UUO with intact contralateral kidney may be because GFR is atypically preserved in the setting of distal tubular damage such that the kidney filters a normal volume but there is limited free water reabsorption. Or this can occur when a pronounced aquaporin channel defect may be present, causing diminished free water absorption in this setting. The diuresis after relief of obstruction is a normal physiologic response to the volume expansion and solute accumulation occurring during obstruction, wherein sodium, urea, and free water are eliminated and the diuresis subsides after solute and fluid homeostasis is achieved. Pathological postobstructive diuresis occurs due to derangement of the medullary solute gradient and downregulation of sodium transporters with subsequent impaired sodium reabsorption in the thick ascending limb of the Henle loop resulting in inappropriate renal handling of water or solutes. Moreover, this can also occur because of poor responsiveness of the collecting duct to antidiuretic hormone (ADH) probably due to a downregulation of aquaporin water channels in this segment of the nephron and perhaps in the proximal tubule.

Q7. Answer E

The development of vasculitis in the adventitial vessels leading to the release of antigens from atheromatous plaque such as ceroid, a complex lipoprotein, which induces an autoimmune antigenic response. The reported inflammatory conditions associated with RPF are IBD, ascending lymphangitis, asbestosis, amyloidosis and sarcoidosis. The classic radiologic findings of medial deviation of extrinsically compressed ureters can be demonstrated in up to 18% of normal subjects. CT reveals a well-defined mass, isodense with muscle in plain films. Tamoxifen is a nonsteroidal anti-oestrogen and is suggested to alter TGF-β, thereby limiting fibrosis. E. F. van Bommel reported a response rate of 74% in patients treated with Tamoxifen 20 mg OD for median duration of 8.5 months.

Q8. Answer B

The reported occurrence of hydronephrosis of pregnancy is between 43% and 100% (Faundes et al. 1998), the wide variation being due to different values used to report hydronephrosis. The right kidney becomes hydronephrotic two to three times more commonly than the left, probably because of interposition of sigmoid colon. Around one third of patients may have persistent hydronephrosis during the first postpartum week, but it resolves within 6 weeks in the majority. Despite the lack of solid evidence, MRI is not advocated in the first trimester of pregnancy (Leyendecker et al. 2004) and gadolinium contrast should be avoided in pregnant patients because it is known to cross the placental barrier. The presence of hydroureter upto the pelvic brim is readily apparent on T2 sequences and is characteristic of this condition. The majority of patients with symptomatic hydronephrosis of pregnancy can be managed with conservative measures. Rapid stent encrustation may be problematic, as urinary calcium excretion increases during pregnancy.

Q9. Answer B

The concentration product, the point at which the dissolved and crystalline components are in equilibrium for a specific set of conditions, at the point of saturation is called the *thermodynamic solubility product*, Ksp. Inhibitors can generally prevent the process of crystal growth or aggregation above the *formation product*, Kf.

Q10. Answer C

Q11. Answer A

Tamm-Horsfall protein, which is the most abundant urinary protein, is secreted by renal epithelial cells in the thick ascending limb and the distal convoluted tubule as a membrane-anchored protein. It is a potent inhibitor of calcium oxalate monohydrate crystal aggregation, but not growth. Nephrocalcin, an acidic glycoprotein, is synthesised in the proximal renal tubules and the thick ascending limb. Osteopontin, or uropontin, is an acidic phosphorylated glycoprotein expressed in bone matrix and renal epithelial cells of the ascending limb of the loop of Henle and the distal tubule. Glycosaminoglycans, acid mucopolysaccharides, and RNA are examples of polyanions that have been shown to inhibit crystal nucleation and growth. The inhibitory activity of magnesium is derived from its complexation with oxalate, which reduces ionic oxalate concentration and calcium oxalate supersaturation. Among the glycosaminoglycans, heparin sulfate interacts most strongly with calcium oxalate monohydrate crystals.

Q12. Answer C

RTA type I, also called 'classic RTA' or 'distal RTA' is the most common form in which the underlying problem is failure of H^+ secretion in the distal nephron. The acquired causes are listed above. The hallmark of the condition is a hyperchloremic metabolic acidosis with a high urinary pH (>5.5) in the face of persistently low serum HCO_3. Patients can also get hypokalemia associated with secondary hyperaldosteronism. These patients are recurrent stone formers mainly composed of calcium phosphate. While sodium bicarbonate corrects the sodium deficit, potassium citrate can increase the citrate levels and prevent stone formation.

Q13. Answer E

Substances like nitric oxide, carbon monoxide, acetylcholine and glucocorticoids decrease the renal artery tone. Vascular tone of the renal blood vessels is the net balance of all these substances and is crucial to the maintenance of GFR, tubular renal function and systemic blood pressure.

Q14. Answer C

Ethanol ingestion and phenytoin inhibit the release of ADH while nicotine and morphine stimulate the release. ADH is released in response to stimulation of osmoreceptor and/or baroreceptors in the carotid sinus and aortic arch. Osmoreceptor stimulation is involved in maintaining tonicity of body fluids. Baroreceptor stimulation leads to renal water retention though increased permeability of the collecting ducts, leading to concentrated urine.

Q15. Answer D

Hyperkalemia could result due to primary renal tubular potassium secretory defect as in sickle-cell disease, systemic lupus erythematosus, postrenal transplantation, obstructive uropathy, tubulointerstitial renal disease and pseudohypoaldosteronism. It can also occur due to inhibition of tubular secretion caused by drugs such as diuretics (amiloride, spironolactone and triamterene), cyclosporine and lithium. Impairment of renin-aldosterone axis can also result in hyperkalemia. Examples of this situation include Addison disease, primary hypoaldosteronism and could be drug induced (heparin, prostaglandin inhibitors, ACE inhibitors, pentamidine and beta blockers) (Leyendecker et al. 2004).

Q16. Answer C

Retroperitoneal fibrosis appears as a fibrous, whitish plaque that encases the aorta, inferior vena cava, and their major branches, and also the ureters and other retroperitoneal structures. An underlying malignancy should always be considered as some report to be present in 8%–10%. Other causes include primary (idiopathic), infections such as tuberculosis, drugs including beta blockers, methyldopa, methysergide, hydralazine, haloperidol, phenacetin pergolide, bromocriptine and ergotomines. Previous radiation or surgical treatment to the abdomen and pelvis has also been implicated. MRI allows superior soft tissue discrimination and can more accurately distinguish the plaque from the great vessels than unenhanced CT. If there is evidence of obstructive uropathy at presentation, therapy should be first directed at its correction. Biopsy to exclude malignancy should be performed next. This can be attempted percutaneously with CT, MRI or ultrasound guidance.

Q17. Answer E

The diagnosis of AKI secondary to AIN may be suggested by the urinalysis findings of sterile pyuria, white blood cell casts and eosinophiluria (using Hansel stain). The clinical presentation usually involves an abnormal urine sediment (described earlier), fever, a rising serum creatinine along with abnormal urinalysis. While skin rash is seen in about 25% of cases, eosinophilia and eosinophiluria are present in more than 75% of cases except in AIN secondary to NSAIDs, where fever, rash and eosinophilia are typically absent. Proteinuria with most drugs is usually modest, with less than 0.5–1 g/day, while in the nephrotic range is frequently seen in selected cases on ampicillin, rifampin, ranitidine and interferon.

EMQs – ANSWERS

Q18. Answer A

Q19. Answer B

Q20. Answer A

Q21. Answer B

Q22. Answer C

Q23. Answer C

Q24. Answer A

Q25. Answer A

Q26. Answer B

The underlying problem of hypernatremia is a disorder of urine concentration with inadequate water intake. This clinical condition is common in the extremes of age. In hypernatremia it is the water balance that matters, and total body sodium can be high, normal, or even low. Treatment of hypernatremia is directed at correction of fluid deficit, water replacement and reversal of underlying causes. Hypovolemia should be initially corrected with half-normal saline. If the patient is awake and not symptomatic, oral hydration with water is sufficient. Otherwise, intravenous (IV) therapy should be started with the goal of slowly lowering plasma osmolality to no more than 2 mOsm/L/hr to avoid cerebral edema. The water deficit can be calculated as

(Volume of distribution) × body weight (kg) × (plasma [Na]/140 − 1). In men, the volume of distribution is 0.5 for men and 0.6 for women.

Q27. Answer A

Q28. Answer B

Q29. Answer C

Q30. Answer D

Q31. Answer D

Q32. Answer C

Q33. Answer A

Cyclosporine causes hypercholesterolaemia, hypertension, gum hypertrophy, constipation, hirsutism and acne. Tacrolimus is a more powerful immunosuppressive than cyclosporine, as indicated by its more potent prophylaxis of transplant rejection. However, its use is associated with diabetes, neurological side effects (tremor, headache), hair loss, gastrointestinal side-effects (e.g., diarrhoea, nausea, vomiting) and hypomagnesaemia. In combination with a myco-phenolate, it may also more often cause over-immunosuppression, namely polyoma nephritis. The mycophenolates inhibit inosinemonophosphate dehydrogenase. This is the rate-limiting step for the synthesis of guanosine monophosphate in the de novo purine pathway.

Q34. Answer A

Q35. Answer C

Q36. Answer E

Q37. Answer D

Q38. Answer F

Q39. Answer B

Q40. Answer F

Sorafenib is an oral multikinase inhibitor with activity against Raf-1 serine/threonine kinase, B-Raf, vascular endothelial growth factor receptor-2 (VEGFR-2), platelet-derived growth factor receptor (PDGFR), FMS-like tyrosine kinase 3 (FLT-3) and c-KIT. Sunitinib is an oxindol tyrosine kinase (TK) inhibitor. It selectively inhibits PDGFR, VEGFR, c-KIT and FLT-3 and has antitumour and anti-angiogenic activity. Pazopanib is an oral angiogenesis inhibitor that targets VEGFR, PDGFR, and c-KIT. Tivozanib is a new oral selective tyrosine kinase inhibitor targeting all three VEGF receptors. Bevacizumab is a humanised monoclonal antibody that binds isoforms of VEGF-A. Temsirolimus is a specific inhibitor of mammalian target of rapamycin (mTOR).

Q41. Answer A

Q42. Answer B

Q43. Answer B

Q44. Answer A

Q45. Answer A

Q46. Answer A

Q47. Answer B

Q48. Answer A

Q49. Answer B

The anion gap is defined as the difference between the levels of routinely measured cations (Na^+) and anions (Cl^- and CO_2) in blood. It is calculated using the formula: Anion gap = $Na^+-(Cl^- + HCO_3^-)$ = 140 – (105 + 24) = 11. The normal range is 9 – 14 mEq/L. The predominant unmeasured anions include albumin, and phosphate. The major unmeasured cations include calcium, magnesium and gamma globulins. If the anion gap is elevated in a patient with metabolic acidosis, the condition occurs because acids that do not contain chloride are present in the blood.

Q50. Answer D

Q51. Answer B

Q52. Answer B

Q53. Answer A

Q54. Answer A

Q55. Answer C

Q56. Answer D

Alkylating agents, like carboplatin, cisplatin, mechlorethamine, cyclophosphamide, chlorambucil, ifosfamide, have the ability to alkylate nucleophilic functional groups under conditions present in cells. They impair cell function by forming covalent bonds with the amino, carboxyl, sulfhydryl, and phosphate groups in biologically important molecules. They work by chemically modifying a cell's DNA. Anti-metabolites act as purines (azathioprine, mercaptopurine) or pyrimidines and prevent them from becoming incorporated into DNA during the 'S' phase (of the cell cycle) and thus stopping normal development and division. They also affect RNA synthesis. Due to their efficiency, these drugs are the most widely used cytostatics. Vinca alkaloids and taxanes are derived from plants and block cell division by preventing microtubule function, which are vital for cell division.

Q57. Answer G, Papillary renal cell cancer

Q58. Answer B, 5 alpha reductase deficiency

Q59. Answer B, Cystinuria

Q60. Answer F, Autosomal dominant polycystic kidney disease

Q61. Answer D, Autosomal recessive polycystic kidney disease

Q62. Answer A, Tuberous sclerosis

Autosomal dominant polycystic kidney disease (ADPKD) is the most common hereditary cystic kidney diseases with an incidence of 1–2:1,000 live births. About 10% of end-stage renal disease (ESRD) patients being treated with hemodialysis were originally diagnosed as ADPKD. There are three genetic mutations in the PKD-1, PKD-2, and PKD3 gene with similar phenotypical presentations. Gene PKD-1 is located on chromosome 16 and codes for a protein involved in the regulation of cell cycle and intracellular calcium transport in epithelial cells, and is responsible for 85% of the cases of ADPKD. A group of voltage-linked calcium channels are coded for by PKD-2 on chromosome 4. The incidence of autosomal recessive polycystic kidney disease (ARPKD) is 1:20,000 live births and is typically identified in the first few weeks after birth. Unfortunately, resulting hypoplasia results in a 30% death rate in neonates with ARPKD.

Tuberous Sclerosis (TSC) is caused by a mutation of either of two genes, TSC1 and TSC2, which code for the proteins hamartin and tuberin, respectively. These proteins act as tumour growth suppressors, agents that regulate cell proliferation and differentiation.

Cystinuria is caused by mutations in the *SLC3A1* and *SLC7A9* genes. These genes encode two parts of a transporter protein that is made primarily in the kidneys. These defects prevent proper reabsorption of basic, or positively charged, amino acids: lysine, ornithine and arginine.

Q63. Answer D

Q64. Answer D

Q65. Answer A

Q66. Answer A

Q67. Answer E

Q68. Answer B

Bicalutamide is an oral non-steroidal pure anti-androgen, which acts by binding to the androgen receptor (AR) and preventing the activation of the AR and subsequent upregulation of androgen responsive genes by androgenic hormones. AFP is a glycoprotein of 591 amino acids with a carbohydrate moiety. Goserelin is a synthetic analogue of a naturally occurring luteinising hormone-releasing hormone (LHRH). Goserelin is poorly protein bound and has a serum elimination half-life of two to four hours in patients with normal renal function. The most common adverse effects of sildenafil use included headache, flushing, dyspepsia, nasal congestion and impaired vision, including photophobia and blurred vision. The half-lives of tadalafil, sildenafil and vardenafil are 17.50 hours, 4.0–5.0 hours, and 4.0–5.0 hours respectively. AFP and BHCG are tumour markers for testicular cancer. AFP has a half-life of 5–7 days, whilst BHCG has a half-life of 24–36 hours.

REFERENCES

1. Faúndes A, Brícola-Filho M, and Pinto e Silva JL. Dilatation of the urinary tract during pregnancy: Proposal of a curve of maximal caliceal diameter by gestational age. *American Journal of Obstetrics and Gynecology* (1998) 178(5): 1082–1086.
2. Leyendecker JR, Gorengaut V, and Brown JJ. MR imaging of maternal diseases of the abdomen and pelvis during pregnancy and the immediate postpartum period. *Radiographics* (2004) 24(5): 1301–1316. Review.

CHAPTER 3: BASIC SCIENCE AND MOLECULAR ONCOLOGY

Paul Cleaveland, Vijay Sangar and Noel Clarke

MCQs

Q1. Which of the following is a neoplastic condition in which malignant cells have not invaded across the cellular basement membrane?
A. Metaplasia
B. Adenocarcinoma
C. Atypical small acinar proliferation
D. Carcinoma in situ
E. Perineural invasion

Q2. At which point of the cell cycle is p53 partially responsible for detecting genetic damage?
A. G1 phase
B. S phase
C. G2/Mitosis checkpoint
D. Mitosis
E. G1/S Checkpoint

Q3. Which of the following represents a premalignant process where abnormal cytological and architectural changes lead to disordered growth and maturation of a cell?
A. Teratoma
B. Metaplasia
C. Dysplasia
D. Atrophy
E. Hyperplasia

Q4. Which of the following is NOT classically related to the effect of radiation therapy on tumour tissue?
A. Radiosensitivity
B. Repair of the cell
C. Hybridisation
D. Reoxygenation
E. Repopulation

Q5. Which one of the following is FALSE regarding apoptosis?
A. It causes cellular shrinkage.
B. It results in the breakdown of organelles.
C. Proteins, cytoplasm and organelles are engulfed by autophagosomes.
D. It leads to the condensation of DNA into chromatin.
E. It causes the leakage of cytosol into the extracellular space (blebbing).

Q6. The loss of function of the VHL protein in renal cell carcinoma is mediated by which of the following?
A. Bcl-2
B. Hypoxia-inducible factor alpha
C. Fibroblast growth factor-3
D. Transforming growth factor beta-1
E. Vascular endothelial growth factor

Q7. Which of the following is the CORRECT sequence of steps in a classical haematological metastatic process?
A. Growth, Extravasation & Migration, Arrest, Survival, Intravasation
B. Extravasation & Migration, Arrest, Survival, Intravasation, Growth
C. Intravasation, Arrest, Extravasation & Migration, Survival, Growth
D. Intravasation, Arrest, Survival, Extravasation & Migration, Growth
E. Extravasation & Migration, Arrest, Growth, Survival, Intravasation

Q8. Regarding the following table, which of the following is FALSE?

	Disease present	Disease not present
Test positive	w	x
Test negative	y	z

A. Sensitivity = w/(w + y).
B. Specificity = z/(x + z).
C. Positive predictive value (of positive test) = w/(w + x).
D. Negative predictive value (of negative test) = y/(x + z).
E. The screen positive rate can be calculated from the table.

Q9. Regarding the major histocompatability complex (MHC), which of following is FALSE?

A. MHC Class I molecules are associated with a light chain, beta-2 microglobulin.
B. T lymphocytes are unable to recognise antigens bound to the MHC molecules.
C. MHC is involved in recognising and binding to foreign antigens.
D. MHC Class II molecules are composed of two heavy chains each with two domains.
E. MHC Class III proteins include cytokines.

Q10. Which of the following immunohistochemical features would be associated with an aggressive tumour in bladder cancer?
A. Low p53
B. High E-cadherin
C. High Ki67
D. Low Rb
E. None of the above

EMQs

Q11–15. Chemotherapy drugs used in uro-oncology
A. Cisplatin
B. Docetaxel
C. Mitomycin
D. Bleomycin
E. Gemcitabine
For each of the modes of action listed below, choose the most appropriate chemotherapeutic agent from the list above.

Q11. Is a M-phase mitotic inhibitor

Q12. Is a non-phase specific alkylating agent

Q13. Is a S-phase antimetabolite

Q14. Is derived from fungal culture

Q15. Requires activation by reductive metabolism

Q16–20. Molecular biology techniques
A. Mass spectrometry
B. FISH
C. PET
D. Microarray
E. Comparative genomic hybridisation
For each of the following descriptions, choose the most appropriate technique from the list above.

Q16. Allows the analysis of complex protein mixtures without separation.

Q17. Multiple DNA probe targets are placed on a glass surface and exposed to fluorescently labelled DNA samples.

Q18. Involves DNA probes labelled with biotin that are coupled with avidin-fluorescein isothiocyanate.

Q19. Allows mapping of chromosomal differences between cells without knowing the cytogenetic abnormality.

Q20. Involves trapping of FDG in the cell.

Q21–25. Statistical descriptions
   A. Prevalence
   B. Incidence
   C. NNT
   D. Relative risk reduction
   E. Absolute risk reduction

For each of the following explanations, choose the most appropriate definition from the list above.

Q21. The proportion by which an intervention reduces the event rate compared to the control group.

Q22. The number of new events in a defined population in a given time period.

Q23. The number of events of a given disease in a defined population at a given time point.

Q24. The difference in the rate of events between the control and intervention groups

Q25. 1/Absolute risk reduction.

Q26–30. Statistical methods
   A. Kaplan–Meier plot
   B. Kappa
   C. Chi-squared
   D. Mann–Whitney U test
   E. T-test

For each of the following descriptions, choose the most appropriate statistical term from the list above.

Q26. A parametric test used to compare the means of two groups.

Q27. A non-parametric test to see if there is a significant difference between two sets of data that have come from two different sets of subjects.

Q28. A measure of the level of agreement between two categorical measures.

Q29. The survival of a sample cohort of which the survival estimates are re-calculated when there is a death.

Q30. Association between two categorical variables.

Q31–35. Flow cytometry analysis

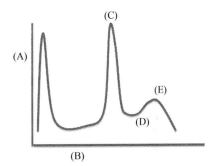

For each of the following, choose the most appropriate part of the flow cytometry curve from the list above.

Q31. S phase

Q32. G2/M phase

Q33. DNA content (Fluorescent intensity)

Q34. G1 peak

Q35. Number of cells

Q36–40. Inherited syndromes associated with malignancy
   A. Von Hippel–Lindau syndrome
   B. Birt–Hogg–Dubé syndrome
   C. Familial papillary renal cell carcinoma
   D. Hereditary leiomyomatosis and renal cell cancer (HLRCC)
   E. Tuberous sclerosis

For each of the following, choose the most answer.

Q36. Associated with epithelioid angiomyolipoma.

Q37. Associated with chromophore renal cell carcinoma.

Q38. Autosomal dominant condition associated with cerebellar haemangioblastomas.

Q39. Mutation in the fumarate hydratase gene.

Q40. Mutation of the c-met proto-oncogene.

Q41–45. Agents used in prostate cancer
   A. Enzalutamide
   B. Docetaxel
   C. Abiraterone acetate
   D. Radium-223
   E. Sipuleucel-T
   F. Strontium-89

For each of the following descriptions, choose the most appropriate technique from the list above.

Q41. Blocks the translocation of the androgen receptor to the cell nucleus.

Q42. Inhibits the 17 alpha-hydroxylase and 17,20-lyase enzymes (CYP17).

Q43. Works through antigen presenting cells to a stimulate T-cell immune response.

Q44. Inhibits depolymerisation of microtubules.

Q45. Is absorbed by metabolically active areas in bone emitting alpha radiation to kill cancer cells.

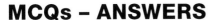

MCQs – ANSWERS

Q1. Answer D

Carcinoma in situ (CIS) is a flat, non-invasive neoplastic condition in which the cancerous cells have not invaded through the basement membrane of the cell. The basement membrane of a cell provides structural support and forms a selective barrier between the cell and the surrounding tissue. Once the cancer cells reach beyond the basement membrane, an invasive neoplasia is formed. In most cancers, CIS is pre-malignant; however, in bladder CIS it is considered to be a pre-invasive papillary cancer in which there is a greater than 50% chance of progression into invasive disease.

Q2. Answer E

DNA damage causes a number of protein-protein interactions that alter protein phosphorylation. Initial sensing of damage is picked up by ATM and ATR proteins. These send signals to phosphorylate CHK2, CHK1, p53, MDM2 and BRCA1, which in turn arrest the cell cycle at checkpoints until DNA damage is repaired. The phosphorylation of p53 proteins causes altered activity in the CDK-inhibitor p21 WAF, which results in G1/S checkpoint arrest. S phase arrest results from phosphorylation of NBS1 and SMC1 directly via ATM. G2/mitosis arrest results from phosphorylation of CDC25C via CHK2 and CHK1.

Q3. Answer C

Dysplasia is a pre-malignant condition where there is abnormal cell growth, cellular atypia and abnormal differentiation. It can be a reversible process in its early stage but once it becomes severe it can progress to neoplasia. Metaplasia a process where one type of differentiated cell transforms into another differentiated cell type. This process is reversible. It is an adaptive response of a tissue to changes in the environment so that the tissue can withstand these changes.

Q4. Answer C

The factors that influence the response of tumour and normal tissue to radiation are known as the 5 R's: radiosensitivity, repair, repopulation, redistribution and reoxygenation. Tumours contain heterogenous cell populations, which vary in their response to radiation. The radiosensitivity, put simply, is the cell kill effect of radiation on a particular type of tissue. The cells ability to repair DNA damage caused by radiation will impact its ability to survive. After or during therapy surviving cells will have the ability to proliferate there by effecting response. A tumour with poor oxygen supply due to inadequate blood supply will be resistant to radiation. After a treatment the tumour blood supply may improve and hence reoxygenation occurs and this improves cell kill effect of further radiation doses. Radiation has differing cell kill effect depending on the cells position within the cell cycle. Radiation results in some synchrony of surviving cells, which then redistribute around the cell cycle. Hybridisation is the fusion of two somatic cells to form a single cell. It can also mean the binding of complimentary sequences of DNA or RNA. This is not classically involved in radiation effect on tumour tissues.

Q5. Answer C

Apoptosis or type 1 cell death is a type of programmed cell death, which is highly regulated and controlled. It is characterised by a sequence of molecular events that lead to particular morphological appearances. These include cellular shrinkage, breakdown of organelles, condensation of DNA into chromatin and blebbing. Autophagic cell death or type 2 cell death is a process where a cell digests itself.

Q6. Answer B

Hypoxia inducible factors are transcription factors that respond to a decrease in oxygen levels on the cellular environment. Inactivation of the VHL protein leads to upregulation of HIF-2 alpha, which in turn leads to upregulation of VEGF, erythropoietin and PEGF. VEGF binds to a tyrosine kinase enzyme (VEGFR-2) on endothelial cells promoting tumour angiogenesis.

Q7. Answer C

The steps of the metastatic process are:

Intravasation – The movement of cells into the blood stream.

Arrest – Cancer cells are larger than most capillaries and hence lodge themselves within the capillaries resulting in arrest.

Extravasation & Migration – Some cells die at the arrest stage but others will pass out of the endothelium into tissue due to the action of cell adhesion molecules, extracellular matrix, growth factors and chemokines.

Survival & Growth – The survival and growth of tumour cells once they are within a particular organ is entirely due to the environment within the organ itself and to the particular tumour cell. Cell-cell, cell-matrix, and growth factor interactions are required for malignant cells to survive and for tumour cells to grow and produce metastatic lesions.

Q8. Answer D

	Disease present	Disease not present
Test positive	w	x
Test negative	y	z

The negative predictive value is calculated as $z/(y + z)$.

The screen positive rate can be calculated as

$$(w + x) / (w + x + y + z).$$

Q9. Answer B

MHC are genes that are found on DNA that code for proteins such as the MHC molecules. T lymphocytes recognise antigens, including tumour antigens, which are bound to MHC molecules on antigen presenting cells.

There are three classes of MHC molecules, I, II and III.

MHC Class I molecules are made up of transmembrane heavy chains (alpha 1, 2 and 3 domains) associated with a light chain, beta-2 microglobulin.

MHC Class II molecules are made of two transmembrane heavy chains each containing two domains, alpha 1/alpha 2 and beta 1/beta 2.

MHC Class III proteins include components of the complement system such as cytokines.

Q10. Answer D

Retinoblastoma (Rb) protein is a tumour suppressor protein, which is involved in preventing excessive cell growth by inhibiting the cell cycle until the point where the cell is ready to divide. At the point of cell division, it is phosphorylated rendering it inactive. p53 is a gene that codes for a protein that regulates the cell cycle and apoptosis. Defective p53 allows abnormal cells to proliferate and lead to cancer. Ki67 is a cellular marker for proliferation, which is associated with ribosomal RNA transcription. Inactivation of Ki67 leads to inhibition of ribosomal RNA synthesis. Increased expression is associated with aggressive pathological features. E-cadherin is a cell adhesion molecule that is involved in adherent junction formation, which allow cells to bind to one another. Decreased expression is associated with increased metastasis.

EMQs – ANSWERS

Q11. Answer B

Q12. Answer A

Q13. Answer E

Q14. Answer D

Q15. Answer C

Cisplatin is an alkylating agent that acts on the rest phase of the cell cycle. It has the ability to crosslink with the purine bases in DNA, thereby interfering with DNA repair mechanisms leading to DNA damage and inducing apoptosis in cancer cells. Docetaxel are plant-derived alkaloids that come from the needles of the European yew tree. It is an anti-microtubular agent, binding to tubulin and inhibiting disassembly. It acts on the M phase of the cell cycle. Mitomycin, derived from streptomyces, requires activation by reduction to produce an alkylating metabolite. Bleomycin is derived from fungal culture. It causes DNA double strand breaks by intercalating with DNA. Gemcitabine is a cytosine analogue. It is converted in the cell to a triphosphate and links to the elongating DNA chain, causing inhibition on DNA synthesis. It acts on the S phase of the cell cycle.

Q16. Answer A

Q17. Answer D

Q18. Answer B

Q19. Answer E

Q20. Answer C

Mass spectrometry generally involves protein sample digestion using trypsin. The resulting peptide mixture is subjected to analysis by electromagnetic chambers that then provide information on the mass charge ratio of each fragment. FISH – fluorescent in situ hybridisation, is undertaken on biopsies or cell cultures, to identify particular areas of DNA. DNA probes are labelled with biotin and are hybridised to chromosomes. The hybridised sequences are picked up using avidin and fluoroscein isothiocyanate, which binds to the biotin. PET – positron emission tomography, allows imaging of a specific biochemical pathway within tissue. FDG ([18F]-fluorodeoxyglucose) is phosphorylated in the cell and becomes trapped within it. The FDG is analysed by a computer and is highlighted. FDG uptake is greater in tumour cells than in normal cells and is therefore used to detect and localise tumours. Microarray involves multiple DNA probe targets being placed on a glass surface and exposed to fluorescently labelled DNA samples. Alternatively different oligo-nucleotide probes are placed on a chip and exposed to DNA samples that are analysed digitally. Comparative genomic hybridisation takes DNA from tumour and benign cells and labels it with two fluorochromes. Conventionally, the tumour DNA is labelled with green fluorescence and the normal with red fluorescence. Changes in DNA are detected by assessing the differences in ratios of the two fluorochromes. This allows the detection of amplification or deletions in chromosomes without knowing the exact cytogenetic abnormality.

Q21. **Answer D**

Q22. **Answer B**

Q23. **Answer A**

Q24. **Answer E**

Q25. **Answer C**

Prevalence is the number of people with a given disease, including new and previously diagnosed, in a specific population, at a given time point. Incidence is the number of events in a defined population over a given time period. NNT – number needed to treat, is the number of people needed to be treated to prevent one bad outcome. This is defined as 1/Absolute risk reduction or (events in control group) – (events in intervention group). Absolute risk reduction is the difference in the rate of events between the control and intervention group. Relative risk reduction is the proportion by which the intervention reduces the event rate. It tells you by how much the treatment reduced the risk of unfavourable outcomes compared to the group that did not have treatment.

Q26. **Answer E**

Q27. **Answer D**

Q28. **Answer B**

Q29. **Answer A**

Q30. **Answer C**

The T-test is a parametric test used to compare the means of two groups. It requires the data to follow a specific distribution and so is used to compare samples of normally distributed data. The Mann–Whitney U test is a non-parametric test of the null hypothesis, which states that there is a significant difference between two sets of data that have come from two different sets of subjects. It is used when data is not normally distributed. Kappa is a statistic that measures how well people or tests agree and is used when data can be put into ordered categories. It is used to see how accurately a test can be replicated. Its value can range for zero to one, where there is no significant agreement to perfect agreement respectively. The Kaplan–Meier plot is a non-parametric statistic used to estimate survival function from lifetime data. It is used to measure the fraction of patients living for a certain period of time after treatment. It is represented as a survival plot and can be used to compare survival between two groups. Chi-squared is a measure of the difference between actual and expected frequencies. The expected frequency is that there is no difference between the sets of results (null hypothesis).

Q31. Answer E

Q32. Answer C

Q33. Answer D

Q34. Answer A

Q35. Answer B

The diagram shows a typical graph from flow cytometry. Flow cytometry allows cells to be sorted depending on DNA content. Cells can be stained with a host of fluorescent markers for various pathways. Hoechst 33342 stains DNA directly. Computer analysis of the fluorescence allows assessment of the amount of DNA in each cell. The graph plots DNA content or fluorescent intensity versus number of cells at the given DNA content. The initial peak shows cell debris. The first peak represents G1 phase and non-proliferating cells. The second peak is G2/M phase, cells that are replicating hence have more DNA within them. The area between these two peaks is S phase, intermediate amounts of DNA.

Q36. Answer E

Q37. Answer B

Q38. Answer A

Q39. Answer D

Q40. Answer C

Von Hippel–Lindau syndrome is an autosomal dominant condition associated with a spectrum of conditions including cerebellar and retinal haemangioblastomas, pancreatic cysts, renal cyst, phaeochromocytomas and renal cell carcinoma. Birt–Hogg–Dubé syndrome is an autosomal dominant condition associated with pulmonary cysts, fibrofolliculomas, oncocytomas, and chromophobe renal cell carcinoma. It is associated with a mutation in the FLCN tumour suppressor gene that codes for follicular on chromosome 17. Familial papillary renal cell carcinoma is an autosomal dominant condition associated with mutation in the c-MET gene on chromosome 7p31. It is associated with type 1 papillary renal cell carcinoma. Hereditary leiomyomatosis and renal cell cancer (HLRCC) is an autosomal dominant condition in which individuals are susceptible to developing cutaneous and uterine leiomyomas as well as type 2 papillary renal cell cancer. It is caused by gremlin mutations in the fumarate hydratase (FH) gene. Tuberous Sclerosis Complex is an autosomal dominant condition characterised by the formation of hamartomas in multiple organs leading to epilepsy, mental retardation and skin manifestations. There is an association with AMLs and renal cell carcinomas. Mutations in TSC1 encoding hamartin and TSC2 encoding tuberin are responsible for the phenotype.

Q41. Answer A

Q42. Answer C

Q43. Answer E

Q44. Answer B

Q45. Answer D

Enzalutamide acts as a selective antagonist and signalling inhibitor of the androgen receptor (AR) leading to its down-regulation. It inhibits the translocation of the AR to the cell nucleus and prevents binding of AR to DNA as well as co-activator proteins. It has a much higher affinity to the AR than other anti-androgens.

Abiraterone inhibits CYP17 enzymes that are expressed in testicular, prostatic and adrenal tissues. The 17-alpha-hydroxylase component catalyses the conversion of pregnenolone and progesterone to their 17-alpha-hydroxy derivatives. 17,20-lyase catalyses the subsequent formation of dehydroepiandrosterone (DHEA) and androstenedione, which are androgens and precursors of testosterone. Abiraterone also acts as a partial AR antagonist.

Sipuleucel-T is an autologous cellular immunological agent. The mechanism of action is unknown; however, it is thought to work through antigen-presenting cells to stimulate a T-cell immune response targeted against prostatic acid phosphatase (an antigen highly expressed in prostate cancer cells).

Docetaxel, a taxane, binds to microtubules and inhibits depolymerisation from calcium ions. This leads to a decrease in free tubulin, which is required for microtubule formation. This results in inhibition of mitotic cell division between metaphase and anaphase.

Radium-223 is an isotope of radium that has a chemical similarity to calcium and is therefore preferentially absorbed by bone. As it decays it emits mainly alpha radiation, which has a short range in tissues producing a localised effect that kills cancer cells. Strontium-89 emits beta radiation to kill cancer cells.

CHAPTER 4: STATISTICS, RESEARCH AND GOVERNANCE

Hamid Abboudi, Erik Mayer and Justin Vale

MCQs

Q1. Which one of the following study designs would be best suited to assess the incidence of secondary pelvic malignancy in patients receiving external beam radiotherapy for prostate cancer?
A. Observational study
B. Randomised controlled study
C. Case-control study
D. Cohort study
E. Cross-sectional study

Q2. In a Kaplan–Meier curve, which term describes removing subjects from the survival analysis who have not completed follow-up at the designated time point?
A. Missing data
B. Listwise deletion
C. Intention to treat
D. Censoring
E. Rounding

Q3. In a non-randomised controlled study evaluating the hypothesis that laparoscopic nephrectomy, as compared with open nephrectomy, reduces the length of hospital stay; the null hypothesis was inappropriately accepted. This is known as?
A. Type I error
B. False positive error
C. Power of a study
D. Publication bias
E. Type II error

Q4. A controlled study, which sequentially allocates consecutive patients to either monopolar TURP or HoLEP to compare short-term outcomes between the two treatment modalities, provides which level of evidence?
A. Level 1
B. Level 2
C. Level 3
D. Level 4
E. Level 5

Q5. In a study evaluating medical therapy for lower urinary tract symptoms, men are randomly allocated to 5-alpha-reductase inhibitor (n = 100) or placebo (n = 100) and subsequently monitored for progression to an episode of acute urinary retention (AUR). In the placebo arm 25 men developed AUR compared with 20 in the 5ARI arm. What is the probability of progressing to AUR in those taking the 5ARI?
A. 0.2
B. 5%
C. 1/4
D. 0.5
E. 25%

Q6. In the same study as described in question 5, what are the odds of developing AUR in the placebo arm?
A. 0.30
B. 0.31
C. 0.32
D. 0.33
E. 0.34

Q7. Publication bias is best detected in a meta-analysis using which of the following graphical forms?
A. Funnel plot
B. Kaplan–Meier curve
C. Receiver operator characteristic curve

D. Forest plot

E. Histogram

Q8. Which of the following statements is INCORRECT when referring to a *p*-value?

A. Assesses the strength of evidence against the null hypothesis.

B. Is the probability that the null hypothesis is true.

C. A *p*-value less than 0.05 means that the 95% confidence interval does not contain the null value.

D. The *p*-value does not indicate the size or importance of the observed effect.

E. When interpreting the results of an analysis, the *p*-value should always be considered alongside the confidence interval.

Q9. A Serious Incident does NOT need to be declared for investigation in which of the following instances?

A. Wrong site surgery

B. Allegation of abuse by a nurse

C. A computer server failure resulting in permanent loss of electronic patient records

D. A multiple trauma patient dying within 24 hours after emergency nephrectomy

E. A retained swab post-operation

Q10. This test is used to compare the medians of two groups of independent non-parametric numerical data

A. Spearman correlation

B. Mann–Whitney U test

C. Chi-square

D. T-test

E. Pearson correlation

EMQs

Q11–16. Statistical terms

A. Absolute risk difference

B. Relative risk ratio

C. Number needed to treat

D. Number needed to harm

E. Prevalence

F. Sensitivity

G. Incidence

H. Negative predictive value

I. Specificity

For each of the descriptions below, choose the most appropriate statistical term from the list above.

Q11. Is calculated as 1 divided by the absolute risk difference

Q12. Is defined as the number of patients who must be treated in order to prevent one adverse event

Q13. Cannot be calculated by a cross-sectional study design

Q14. Is most commonly used to quantify the strength of an association between a risk factor/exposure and a disease/outcome

Q15. Is dependent on the prevalence of the disease in the population

Q16. Is equal to 1 minus the false negative rate

Q17–22. Statistical terms

A. Standard error

B. Mean

C. Interquartile range

D. Median

E. Confidence interval

F. Mode

G. Standard deviation

H. *p*-value

I. Normal distribution

For each of the descriptions below, choose the most appropriate statistical term from the list above.

Q17. Is used along with the median value to draw a box and whisker plot

Q18. Is symmetrical about the mean and bell-shaped

Q19. For a population, measures the variation of individual observations from the mean value

Q20. Is a measure of how closely a sample mean estimates a population mean

Q21. Is most commonly calculated using 1.96 standard errors above and below the population mean

Q22. Is a useful descriptive measure of the average value if a dataset includes extremely high and low values

Q23–28. Research and development terms
A. Clinical effectiveness & research
B. Audit
C. Risk management
D. Education and training
E. Financial and commercial dealings
F. Using information & information technology
G. Staffing & staff management
H. Patient and public involvement

For each of the descriptions below, choose the most appropriate term from the list above.

Q23. Is not typically used to describe one of the seven pillars of clinical governance

Q24. Incorporates the need to maintain confidentiality of patient data

Q25. Includes the practice of evidence-based medicine

Q26. Promotes a blame-free culture and is commonly monitored by a committee chaired by the medical director or CEO

Q27. The annual Record of In-Training Assessments forms a component of this

Q28. Is partly implemented by involvement in the national patient surveys collated by the Care Quality Commission

MCQs – ANSWERS

Q1. Answer D

Sampling in a case-control study is determined by a disease state, not an exposure status. The controls represent the population at risk of the disease (but do not have it) and the cases that have the disease. Case-control studies can either be unmatched (the controls are selected at random from the population at risk) or matched where each case is matched with a control for potential confounding variables. In case-control studies, a form of observational study, subjects are observed and therefore not randomised. Cohort studies contrast with case-control studies in that the subjects are sampled based on their exposure, or not, to a variable of interest and then observed until the outcome being investigated occurs. Cohort studies are therefore an example of a longitudinal study design because subjects are followed over time. Data acquisition can either be prospective or retrospective. Intervention studies, which are another form of longitudinal study, do allow for randomisation of subjects to intervention or treatment groups. Randomised controlled trials (RCTs) are a true experimental study design and provide optimal evidence in healthcare on the effectiveness of treatments/healthcare interventions specific to a population of interest. RCTs should, wherever possible, incorporate some element of 'blinding' of subjects (patients), healthcare providers and/or data collectors to provide the most robust evidence. RCTs should be reported according to the CONSORT statement. A cross-sectional study is a descriptive study and makes estimates of features of the population of interest at a single time point or over a continuous short period of time. It is commonly used to determine prevalence of disease in a population.

Q2. Answer D

A Kaplan–Meier curve is a commonly used analysis to calculate survival after a treatment using lifetime data. Censoring correctly describes the process of removing subjects from a survival analysis if they have not completed follow-up at the stipulated time-point and can be incorporated in a Kaplan–Meier analysis. Intention-to-treat analysis describes an analysis methodology that, instead of removing subjects that deviate from an agreed protocol, includes them all in the final analysis based on their initial treatment intent. Listwise deletion describes removal of a record if a single data item is missing. It is a generic method for handling missing data in statistics and is not particular to Kaplan–Meier analysis. Rounding up or rounding down a figure is commonly used in mathematics to simplify interpretation.

Q3. Answer E

A type I error (or false positive error) is said to have occurred when a null hypothesis, which is true, is inappropriately rejected. The probability of making a type I error is equal to the chosen significance level (p-value). Conversely, when a null hypothesis, which is false, fails to be rejected, a type II error (or false negative error) is said to have occurred. The probability of not making a type II error equals the power of the test. Publication bias is not related to hypothesis testing and statistical error.

Q4. Answer B

The use of levels of evidence, in evidence-based medicine, is a means by which the reader can stratify, in a standardised manner, the evidence according to its quality. A number of systems have been designed for this purpose, including that produced by the Oxford Centre for Evidence-Based Medicine [1]; a modified version of which is used by the European Association of Urology clinical guidelines to formulate its grades of recommendations.

Q5. Answer A

Q6. Answer D

It is important to be able to distinguish between risk (probability) and odds as they are both often used in published studies, but are not interchangeable. The risk, or probability, is defined as the number of subjects experiencing the outcome of interest divided by the total population at risk/being studied. It can either be expressed as a value between 0 (never occurred) to 1 (always occurred) or as a percentage. This contrasts to odds which equals the probability of an event occurring divided by the probability that it does not. Odds and odds ratio (odds in 'exposed' group divided by odds in 'unexposed' group) are often used in studies reporting on binary outcome variables (e.g., mortality).

Q7. Answer A

Funnel plots graphically display a measure of study precision (vertical axis) against treatment effects for each of the studies included in the meta-analysis. The resultant symmetry or indeed asymmetry can give an indication of the presence of publication bias. Publication bias describes the phenomenon whereby systematic reviews and meta-analysis do not necessarily include all available studies of interest; smaller studies without statistically significant results are less likely to be published. In the absence of publication bias, a symmetrical inverted funnel (hence the name funnel plot) is generated because the treatment effect estimates from smaller studies scatter more widely at the base of the graph with those of larger studies narrowing towards the apex. If a meta-analysis is over-represented by larger studies with more significant results, and therefore, smaller studies are not included, asymmetry of the 'funnel' occurs. Funnel plots are commonly used by the Cochrane collaboration reviews. Receiver operator characteristic (ROC) curve is a plot of a test's (with a binary outcome) sensitivity (y-axis) against 1 – specificity (x-axis) using different cut-off values. By calculating the area under the curve, the accuracy (discriminatory ability) of the test can be determined. Forest plots are commonly used in a meta-analysis of randomised controlled trials and is a way of presenting the outcome data for each RCT included in the meta-analysis (including the confidence intervals and weight of each RCT in the meta-analysis) and provides a summary estimate. Histograms are used to illustrate frequency distributions of data.

Q8. Answer B

A p-value is generated by performing a hypothesis (significance) test and provides a measure of how confident one can be in rejecting the null hypothesis. A commonly used cut-off for a statistically significant result is <0.05 and with a p-value below this, the null value will not be within the 95% confidence limits. At this level, there is less than a 5% probability that the observed effect could have resulted by chance if the null hypothesis were true. The confidence interval should always be interpreted alongside the p-value, as even with a very significant result (very low p-value), the confidence interval may indicate no important difference between groups.

Q9. Answer D

Reporting of serious incidents in the NHS should be aligned to the national framework produced by the National Patient Safety Agency 'Serious Incident Reporting and Learning Framework (SIRL)'. This framework was introduced to ensure consistency in definitions of serious incidents, roles and responsibilities and clarify legal and regulatory requirements. A full list of serious incidents requiring investigation are available in the document 'National Framework for Reporting and Learning from Serious Incidents Requiring Investigation'.

Q10. Answer B

Spearman correlation is used to establish an association between non-normally distributed numerical variables. Chi-square is the test that compares the proportion of people with a particular attribute in two or more independent groups of categorical data. T-test is used to compare the means of two groups of parametric numerical data. Pearson correlation is used to determine the strength of a relationship of a continuous normally distributed variable amongst two groups.

EMQs – ANSWERS

Q11. Answer C

Q12. Answer C

Q13. Answer G

Q14. Answer B

Q15. Answer H

Q16. Answer F

Absolute risk reduction (ARR) of a disease is your risk of developing the disease over a time period. The same absolute risk can be expressed in different ways. For example, a 1 in 10 risk of developing a certain disease in your life. This can also be said to be a 10% risk, or a 0.1 risk – depending on whether you use percentages or decimals. Relative risk ratio (RR) is the proportion of bad outcomes in the intervention group divided by the proportion of bad outcomes in the control group. When a treatment has a RR greater than 1, the risk of a bad outcome is increased by the treatment; when the RR is less than 1, the risk of a bad outcome is decreased, meaning that the treatment is likely to do good. When the RR is exactly 1, the risk is unchanged.

The Number Needed to Treat is the number of patients who need to be treated to prevent one additional bad outcome (e.g., the number of patients that need to be treated for one of them to benefit compared with a control). It is defined as the inverse of the absolute risk reduction (NNT = 1/ARR).

Prevalence is the proportion of cases in the population at a given time and therefore indicates how widespread the disease is. Incidence is the rate of occurrence of new cases. Thus, incidence conveys information about the risk of contracting the disease.

Sensitivity refers to the proportion of true positives correctly identified by the test.

Specificity refers to the proportion of true negatives correctly identified by the test.

Positive predictive value is the proportion of those who test positive who actually have the disease. Whilst negative predictive value is the proportion of those who test negative who actually do not have the disease.

Q17. Answer C

Q18. Answer I

Q19. Answer G

Q20. Answer A

Q21. Answer E

Q22. Answer D

Standard error is a measure of how closely a sample mean estimates a population mean whereas the standard deviation of the sample is the degree to which individuals within the sample differ from the sample mean.

The mean is obtained by dividing the sum of all values by the total number of values and hence is greatly influenced by very high values.

The interquartile range is the observation corresponding to the 25th centile to the observation corresponding to the 75th centile and will contain 50% of the data. Its value is unaffected by the top 25% and the bottom 25% of data values.

The median is the value that comes halfway when the data are ranked, whilst the mode is the value that occurs most frequently.

The confidence interval (CI) contains information about the (im) precision of the estimated effect size. It presents a range of values, on the basis of the sample data, in which the population value for such an effect size may lie. If the CI includes zero, the study has given evidence that no effect of treatment is feasible.

p-Value is the probability of how true the null hypothesis is using evidence provided by the observed data. A $p \leq 0.05$ suggests a 5% probability that the null hypothesis is true and is commonly used as a cut-off for statistical significance.

Q23. Answer E

Q24. Answer F

Q25. Answer A

Q26. Answer C

Q27. Answer D

Q28. Answer H

Clinical governance provides a framework through which NHS organisations are accountable for continually improving quality of their services and safeguarding high standards of care by creating an environment in which excellence in clinical care will flourish [2]. Clinical governance has been described using 7 key pillars: clinical effectiveness and research (evidence based approach, implementing guidelines), audit, risk management (robust systems in place to understand, monitor and minimise risks to patients), education and training (courses, conferences, exams and appraisal), patient and public involvement (local patient feedback, patient advice and liaison service) using information and IT (accurate patient data and confidentiality) and staffing and staff management (recruitment, management, retention of staff and providing good working conditions).

REFERENCES

1. Oxford Centre for Evidence-Based Medicine Levels of Evidence, (May 2009). Produced by Bob Phillips, Chris Ball, Dave Sackett, Doug Badenoch, Sharon Straus, Brian Haynes, Martin Dawes since November 1998. Updated by Jeremy Howick March 2009. www.cebm.net

2. G Scally and L J Donaldson, Clinical governance and the drive for quality improvement in the new NHS in England, *BMJ* (4 July 1998): 61–65.

CHAPTER 5: IMAGING AND PRINCIPLES OF URO-RADIOLOGY

Anuj Goyal, Beth Hickerton and Rebecca Tregunna

MCQs

Q1. Which of the following statements about diagnostic ultrasonography is INCORRECT?
   A. At lower ultrasound frequencies, there is better penetration but worse resolution.
   B. At higher ultrasound frequencies, there is worse penetration but better resolution.
   C. Acoustic impedance influences the amount of energy reflected from tissue interfaces.
   D. Diagnostic medical ultrasound frequencies are typically between 2 and 18 KHz, which is above the audible range of normal human hearing.
   E. Fat appears echo-bright on ultrasound.

Q2. During a CT for abdominal trauma which of the following statements is INCORRECT?
   A. The arterial phase is captured 25 seconds after intravenous contrast injection.
   B. 150 mL of Omnipaque may be used as the contrast agent, injected at 3 mL/second.
   C. The venous phase is captured at 10 to 15 minutes after intravenous contrast injection.
   D. Images are obtained in 1 mm or 2.5 mm slices.
   E. Delayed phase (excretory phase) is required to grade renal trauma.

Q3. In relation to an emergency on-table IVU, which of the following is INCORRECT?
   A. It is most appropriate during a laparotomy to provide detail of renal injury.
   B. An intravenous bolus of iodinated contrast at 2 mL/kg body weight is used.
   C. It is most appropriate during laparotomy to provide detail of a functioning contralateral kidney.
   D. Involves a single shot KUB X-ray at 10 minutes following administration of contrast.
   E. It is preferable not to use fluoroscopy screening due to poor quality images.

Q4. Which of the following statements is INCORRECT?
   A. Foetal death during general anaesthetic is most likely in the second trimester of pregnancy.
   B. Ultrasound with Doppler can be used to investigate renal colic by assessing for the presence of ureteral jets.
   C. A limited IVU is considered safe in pregnancy.
   D. Ureteroscopy and holmium laser stone fragmentation has been used safely to treat urinary tract stones during pregnancy when treatment cannot be delayed.
   E. Obstruction secondary to ureteric stones during pregnancy can be managed with analgesia and a nephrostomy.

Q5. Which of the following statements is INCORRECT?
   A. T1-weighted MRI images show water to be dark.
   B. T2-weighted MRI images show water to be bright.
   C. Gadolinium uptake in tissues makes them appear brighter on T1-weighted MRI images.
   D. Neutrons in the nucleus of the hydrogen atom have a negative charge.
   E. Gadolinium should not be given if eGFR is less than 30 mL/min/1.73 m^2 due to risk of nephrogenic systemic fibrosis.

Q6. Which of the following statements about multi-parametric prostate MRI is TRUE?

A. Malignant areas within the prostate have a high signal intensity on T2-weighted MRI.

B. There are increased levels of citrate in cancerous prostatic tissue on MR spectroscopy.

C. There are increased levels of choline in cancerous prostatic tissue on MR spectroscopy.

D. Multiparametric MRI does not employ gadolinium-based contrast therefore it is a safe test in patients with renal failure.

E. The T2-weighted sequence can be regarded as a functional form of imaging.

Q7. Which of the following statements is INCORRECT?

A. Clear cell renal cell carcinoma generally appears hyperintense on T2-weighted MRI.

B. Simple renal cysts appear hyperintense on T1-weighted MRI.

C. MRI is better than CT when assessing for the extent of a venous tumour thrombus.

D. The main MRI feature indicating potential malignancy in a renal mass is contrast enhancement.

E. Oncocytomas show a variable low to moderate signal intensity on T1-weighted MR images.

Q8. All of the following agents can be used for a dynamic renography study, except:

A. ^{123}Iodine-labelled ortho-iodohippurate

B. ^{99m}Technetium-labelled dimercaptosuccinic acid

C. ^{99m}Technetium-labelled diethylene triamine pentaacetic acid

D. ^{99m}Technetium-labelled mercaptoacetyltriglycine

E. ^{99m}Technetium-labelled ethylene dicysteine

Q9. Which of the following statements about a ^{99m}Technetium-labelled dimercaptosuccinic acid (^{99m}Tc-DMSA) renogram is correct?

A. 10% of ^{99m}Tc-DMSA is taken up by active proximal convoluted tubular cells.

B. 90% of ^{99m}Tc-DMSA is excreted in the urine by tubular secretion.

C. One-third of the injected ^{99m}Tc-DMSA radio-isotope is renal bound within one hour.

D. Is significantly more accurate than a ^{99m}Tc-MAG-3 renogram for assessing differential renal function.

E. ^{99m}Tc-DMSA renograms in adults deliver a total effective radiation dose of 0.3 mSv.

Q10. Which of the following statements about bone scans performed to detect metastatic malignancy is correct?

A. ^{99m}Technetium-labelled methylene diphosphonate (^{99m}Tc-MDP) has high skeletal affinity and poor blood clearance.

B. Images are obtained at 60 minutes following intravenous injection of the radioisotope.

C. Patients are asked not to void prior to imaging.

D. False negatives results may occur in metastatic deposits of aggressive anaplastic tumours.

E. Bone scans help detect metastatic bone deposits by the increased osteoclastic activity they induce.

Q11. Which of the following statements in relation to dual energy *X-ray* absorptiometry (DEXA) scans is CORRECT?

A. An initial DEXA T-score of below −2.5 is considered low risk and no further scanning is required in patients receiving ADT for prostate cancer.

B. An initial DEXA T-score between −1 and −2.5 is classified as intermediate risk in patients receiving ADT for prostate cancer and requires further DEXA scans every year.

C. Risk of sustaining a bone fracture after five years of androgen deprivation therapy is 50%.

D. DEXA scans are whole body scans and are safe in pregnancy.

E. A DEXA scan requires approximately 90 minutes scan time.

Q12. Which of the following statements is TRUE?

A. Iodinated intravenous ionic contrast agents are safer than the non-ionic types.

B. Gadolinium-based contrast is safe in severe renal failure.

C. Metformin must be stopped prior to the use of any iodinated intravenous contrast.

D. Nephrogenic systemic fibrosis is a recognised side effect following use of gadolinium-based contrast agents.

E. Anaphylaxis to a contrast agent is treated with 5 mg intravenous 1:1000 adrenaline.

Q13. Regarding telescopes as used in cystoscopy, which of the following statements is true?

A. A 70° telescope has a yellow band on its light connector to help identify it.

B. A 30° telescope has a green band on its light connector to help identify it.

C. The 'Hopkins Rod-Lens System' consists of short glass rods separated by longer gaps of air.

D. The 'Hopkins Rod-Lens System' uses the concept of total internal reflection for the transmission of light.

E. Cystoscopes range from 25 to 28 French in size.

EMQs

Q14–19. What imaging frequencies and radiation doses apply for the following imaging modalities?

A. 3.5 MHz
B. 7 MHz
C. 12 MHz
D. 0.02 mSv
E. 6.3 mSv
F. 4.7 mSv
G. 15 mSv
H. 2.5 mSv

For each of the following descriptions, select the most appropriate answer from the list above. Each option may be used once, more than once or not at all.

Q14. Diagnostic renal ultrasound

Q15. Radiation dose of a CT urogram

Q16. Bone scan radiation dose

Q17. CT KUB radiation dose

Q18. IVU radiation dose

Q19. Transrectal ultrasound probe for evaluation of the prostate gland

Q20–25. Which imaging modality would be first line in the investigation of the following scenarios?

A. CT Urogram
B. Non-contrast CT KUB
C. A CT scan from the head to thighs with imaging sequences obtained at 25 seconds, 60 seconds, 10–15 minutes, along with a CT cystogram
D. USS kidneys
E. IVU
F. Resuscitation, surgical exploration of the injury with a one-shot on-table IVU in theatre
G. USS testes
H. Imaging not indicated
I. CT chest, abdomen and pelvis

For each of the following descriptions, select the most appropriate answer from the list above. Each option may be used once, more than once or not at all.

Q20. A 50-year-old woman with an 8-hour history of severe colicky left loin pain and microscopic haematuria

Q21. A 38-year-old haemodynamically stable man with right-sided abdominal pain and visible haematuria following a mountain bike accident

Q22. A 23-year-old male with a 2-hour history of acute-onset testicular pain

Q23. A 46-year-old haemodynamically unstable man with a penetrating injury to the right loin following a road traffic accident

Q24. A 50-year-old man with visible haematuria and a normal flexible cystoscopy

Q25. A 73-year-old lady with a solid-looking bladder tumour on flexible cystoscopy

Q26–31. What is the MOST appropriate modality of imaging in the following scenarios concerning the management of prostate cancer?
  A. X-ray pelvis
  B. Bone scan and multiparametric MRI prostate
  C. DEXA scan
  D. MRI whole spine
  E. CT spine
  F. ^{11}C-Choline PET
  G. Bone scan alone
  H. Multiparametric MRI prostate
  I. MRI lumbar spine

For each of the following descriptions, select the most appropriate answer from the list above. Each option may be used once, more than once or not at all.

Q26. An 84-year-old male with Gleason 3 + 4 prostate cancer, PSA 13 at diagnosis, with a stable PSA of 5.4, controlled on LHRH analogues for 12 years

Q27. A 76-year-old male with known prostate cancer (Gleason 4 + 5) presenting with severe lower back pains and difficulty walking

Q28. A 54-year-old gentleman with a newly diagnosed Gleason 4 + 4 = 8 adenocarcinoma of the prostate gland in 2 biopsy cores, with a presenting PSA of 21 and being considered for radical treatment

Q29. An asymptomatic 88-year-old man with a T4 feeling prostate and a PSA of 15

Q30. A 50-year-old man with negative biopsies of the prostate and a rising PSA

Q31. A 64-year-old man four years post radical prostatectomy for pT2a N0Gleason 3 + 4 = 7 prostate cancer with a PSA of 1.1 ng/mL and rising

Q32–37. Which is the CORRECT laser type for use in urology which matches to the following statements?
  A. Kalium titanyl phosphate (KTP:Nd:YAG)
  B. Holmium (Ho:YAG)
  C. Neodymium (Nd:YAG)
  D. CO_2
  E. Thulium (Tm:YAG)
  F. Argon
  G. Diode
  H. Lithium Borate (LBO:Nd:YAG)

For each of the following descriptions, select the most appropriate answer from the list above. Each option may be used once, more than once or not at all.

Q32. Has a wavelength of 2140 nm

Q33. Has a wavelength of 532 nm

Q34. Has a wavelength of 1064 nm

Q35. Used for green light laser vaporisation of the prostate gland

Q36. Most commonly used laser for stone fragmentation during ureteroscopy

Q37. Has a tissue penetration depth of 3–5 mm and used to ablate early penile cancers

Q38–40. In these trauma scenarios what is the MOST appropriate form of imaging?
  A. CT abdomen and pelvis and a CT cystogram
  B. CT abdomen and pelvis
  C. CT chest, abdomen and pelvis
  D. USS KUB
  E. KUB X-ray
  F. Retrograde urethrogram, +/− catheterisation and a delayed CT abdomen and pelvis +/− cystogram
  G. Retrograde urethrogram
  H. IVU

For each of the following descriptions, select the most appropriate answer from the list above. Each option may be used once, more than once or not at all.

Q38. A 28-year-old female with frank haematuria and pelvic pain following a fall from a horse

Q39. A conscious and haemodynamically stable biker following a road traffic accident with blood at his external urethral meatus

Q40. A 35-year-old man with a history of a cracking sound during sexual intercourse followed by immediate detumescence and inability to void

Q41–44. Which commonly used laboratory stains are used diagnostically for the following conditions?
A. Haematoxylin and eosin staining
B. Ziehl–Neelsen staining
C. Gram stain
D. Papanicolaou staining
E. Nucleic acid amplification test (NAAT)
F. Hale's colloidal iron stain

For each of the following descriptions, select the most appropriate answer from the list above. Each option may be used once, more than once or not at all.

Q41. Tuberculosis

Q42. Chlamydia

Q43. Urine cytology

Q44. Chromophobe renal cell carcinoma

Q45–48. Which answer corresponds to the following statements concerning diathermy?
A. Monopolar
B. CUT
C. Voltage
D. COAG
E. Bipolar
F. Alternating current
G. Power

For each of the following descriptions, select the most appropriate answer from the list above. Each option may be used once, more than once or not at all.

Q45. Continuous, high-power, low-voltage waveform

Q46. Pulsed, low-power, high-voltage waveform

Q47. Force that enables the electrons to move around an electrical circuit

Q48. Measured in units of watts

Q49–52. Concerning the principles of decontamination and sterilisation which of the following applies to the statements below?
A. Contamination
B. Decontamination
C. Cleaning
D. Disinfection
E. Sterilisation

For each of the following descriptions, select the most appropriate answer from the list above. Each option may be used once, more than once or not at all.

Q49. A validated process used to render a product free from viable microorganisms

Q50. Level of cleaning required for flexible cystoscopes before use in a patient

Q51. Effect of chlorine dioxide

Q52. Effect of steam cleaning at 121°C for 15 minutes

Q53–56. The following endoluminal instruments are commonly of which French gauge (Fr) in size?
A. 0.038 Fr
B. 3 Fr
C. 4.7 Fr
D. 7 Fr
E. 22 Fr
F. 28 Fr

For each of the following descriptions, select the most appropriate answer from the list above. Each option may be used once, more than once or not at all.

Q53. Resectoscope

Q54. Standard guide wire

Q55. Semi-rigid ureteroscope

Q56. Cystoscope

MCQs – ANSWERS

Q1. Answer D

Ultrasound can be used as a diagnostic medical imaging technique that utilises the interaction between sound waves and different tissues. Alternative current is applied to crystals of a piezo-ceramic plate in a transducer. Expansion and contraction of these crystals produce longitudinal waves, typically at a frequency varying between 2 and 18 MHz. In humans, the audible range of sound wave frequency is between 20 and 20,000 Hz. As the sound waves travel through tissues some are reflected back and are converted from their mechanical form to electrical energy by the transducer to produce an image.

Artefacts occur due to acoustic shadowing, distal enhancement, edging and reverberation.

Q2. Answer C

An emergency CT needs to be discussed with a radiologist, with a responsible doctor involved in the transfer of the patient if stable enough to undergo imaging. Prior to the emergency CT, the patient needs a urinary catheter and an intravenous cannula in place. 150 mL of intravenous iodinated contrast such as Omnipaque should be injected at 3 mL/second. Patients are scanned in a cranio-caudal direction. The arterial phase is captured at 25 seconds and the venous phase at 60 seconds. EAU recommends a delayed abdominal and pelvic scan at 10–15 minutes to visualise the collecting systems in all patients with suspected renal trauma, with or without a cystogram. Images are generally obtained in 2.5-mm slices.

References and Further Reading

Standards of practice and guidance for trauma radiology in severely injured patients, Second Edition. London, UK: The Royal College of Radiologists, 2015.

Q3. Answer A

An emergency on-table IVU will generally only tell you if there is a normally functioning contralateral kidney and is unlikely to provide reliable or adequate detail on the actual injury itself. Two mL/kg of an iodinated contrast agent such as Omnipaque should be administered as a rapid bolus via a large bore cannula, ideally in placed in the antecubital fossa. A single shot KUB X-ray is then obtained at 10 minutes.

Q4. Answer A

Urolithiasis during pregnancy is uncommon. A multidisciplinary team approach must be adopted to include the urologist, obstetrician, anaesthetist and radiologist. The health of the mother and the development of the foetus are paramount. There is however an absence of prospective studies in this area. Ultrasound is the primary radiological investigation of choice, followed by either an MRI or a limited IVU. Fortunately, conservative supportive management will result in the spontaneous passage of the stone in the majority of pregnant patients. The accepted safe cumulative dose of ionizing radiation to the foetus in pregnancy is five rad (50 mGy), and no single diagnostic study should exceed this maximum. The most sensitive time period for central nervous system teratogenesis is between 10 and 17 weeks of gestation. Non-urgent radiological testing should therefore be avoided during this period. Rare consequences of excessive fetal radiation exposure include a slight increase in the incidence of some childhood cancers, such as leukaemias and, possibly, a very small change in the frequency of genetic mutations. When surgical intervention is necessary insertion of a nephrostomy to relieve the obstruction along with analgesia is an option. Ureteroscopy and holmium laser lithotripsy in pregnancy have been shown to be safe in a number of reports. However, these trials include small numbers and there exists some controversy on the possible detrimental effects of intracorporeal lithotripsy on the foetus' hearing.

References and Further Reading

Srirangam B, Hickerton B, and van Cleynenbreugel B. Management of urinary calculi in pregnancy: A review. *Journal of Endourology* (2008) 22(5): 867–875.

Toppenberg KS, Hill DA, and Miller DP. Safety of radiographic imaging during pregnancy. *American Family Physician* (1999) 1;59(7): 1813–1818.

Q5. Answer D

MRI uses the magnetic properties of hydrogen and its interaction with both a large external magnetic field and radio waves to produce highly detailed images of the human body. The nucleus of an atom consists of protons (positive charge) and neutrons (neutral charge). The most common Hydrogen atom isotope in the human body (Protium) has a single proton in its nucleus and no neutrons. The protons are in motion and spin about their axis. When placed in a magnetic field, the protons always align either parallel or anti-parallel to the direction of the magnetic field. When excited by a radio wave they flip direction. Over time, they flip back, emitting a radio signal (MR signal), which is captured by the scanner.

T1 represents longitudinal relaxation time. This indicates the time required for a substance to become magnetised after first being placed in a magnetic field. This involves a transfer of energy. T1-weighted MR images show fat to be bright and water dark. T2 is the transverse relaxation time (decay). It is a measure of how long transverse magnetisation would last in a perfectly uniform external magnetic field. T2-weighted MR images show fluid/water to be bright and fat to be intermediate to dark.

Q6. Answer C

Multiparametric MRI is being used more commonly for the imaging of prostate cancer. This employs various image acquisition formats including diffusion-weighting, dynamic contrast enhancement and MR spectroscopy to provide additional functional information. This increases specificity for the detection of prostatic malignancy. Intravenous gadolinium is used as an enhancing contrast agent. Most prostate cancer occurs in the peripheral zone and can be visualised as low-signal-intensity areas in a background of high-signal intensity produced by normal tissues on T2-weighted MR images. Diffusion weighting shows the extent of random Brownian motion of water molecules within the tissues, thereby providing information on tissue composition and the integrity of membranes. MR Spectroscopy can differentiate between the metabolic levels of tissues. In healthy prostate, there are high levels of citrate and polyamines and decreased levels of choline. This pattern is reversed in prostate cancer. Choline is a marker of cellular proliferation.

Q7. Answer B

The use of MRI in the evaluation of renal abnormalities is increasing. It is particularly useful for investigating patients with compromised renal function, severe allergy to iodinated contrast, or where radiation exposure is to be avoided, such as in children and pregnant women. The signal intensity of simple renal cysts on MRI mirrors that of water, appearing hypointense on T1-weighted images and hyperintense on T2-weighted images. EAU guidelines endorse level 3 evidence for MRI to assess venous involvement if the extent of vena caval thrombus if poorly defined on CT scanning in T3 renal cell carcinoma. The MRI appearances of renal oncocytoma is typically hypointense as compared to normal renal parenchyma on non-enhanced T1-weighted images. They usually exhibit high signal intensity on T2-weighted sequences.

References and Further Reading

Nikken JJ and Krestin GP. MRI of the kidney–state of the art. *European Radiology* (2007) 17(11): 2780–2793.

Q8. Answer B

Renograms are static or dynamic renal scintigraphy studies that employ a radiotracer to study various aspects of renal morphology and function by analysing radiotracer uptake, filtration, secretion and excretion in the kidneys. ^{99m}Technetium-labelled dimercaptosuccinic acid (DMSA) is the agent most commonly used in static renal scintigraphy scans. DMSA is an organosulphur compound that is actively extracted and bound by functioning nephrons; little is filtered. All the other agents listed can be used in dynamic renal scintigraphy studies to provide information on excretion and drainage from the kidney.

Q9. Answer C

Following an intravenous injection of the radiotracer compound, ^{99m}Technetium-labelled dimercaptosuccinic acid static (^{99m}Tc-DMSA) renogram images are obtained with a gamma camera three to four hours later. ^{99m}Tc-DMSA is a protein bound organosulphur compound that is actively extracted and bound by functioning renal tubules and little is filtered. It is avidly taken up by active proximal convoluted cells largely via peri-tubular uptake (approximately two-thirds) and to a lesser extent via glomerular filtration (one-third). It is minimally excreted in the urine by tubular secretion. Approximately one-third of the isotope is renal bound within 1 hour and 50% within 6 hours. The remainder gets sequestered in the liver, spleen and bones. ^{99m}Tc-MAG-3 renogram scans are equally capable of assessing split renal function but ^{99m}Tc-DMSA scans provide excellent additional assessment of renal morphology and evidence of cortical scarring. The total radiation dose from a ^{99m}Tc-DMSA renogram has been shown to be 3.3 mSv.

References and Further Reading

Çelik T, Yalçin H, Günay EC, Özen A, and Özer C. Comparison of the relative renal function calculated with 99mTc-diethylenetriaminepentaacetic acid and 99mTc-dimercaptosuccinic acid in children. *World Journal of Nuclear Medicine* (2014) 13(3): 149–153.

De Lange MJ, Piers DA, Kosterink JG, van Luijk WH, Meijer S, de Zeeuw D, and van der Hem L. Renal handling of technetium-99m DMSA: Evidence for glomerular filtration and peritubular uptake. *Journal of Nuclear Medicine* (1989) 30(7): 1219–1223.

Mettler FA, Huda W, Yoshizumi TT, and Mahesh M. Effective doses in radiology and diagnostic nuclear medicine: A catalog. *Radiology* (2008) 248(1): 254–263.

Q10. Answer D

^{99m}Technecium-labelled methylene diphosphonate (^{99m}Tc-MDP) has high skeletal affinity and rapid blood clearance. 400–800 MBq ^{99m}Tc-MDP (half-life of six hours) is injected into a peripheral vein. There is maximal bone uptake by two hours after injection, but imaging is delayed to take place at three to four hours post injection. This delay permits unbound tracer to be eliminated by the kidneys. Voiding is performed immediately prior to imaging to enable visualisation of the pelvis. Uptake is determined by local blood flow and the level of osteoblastic activity. False positive results may be seen at sites of healing fractures, Paget's disease, osteomyelitis or degenerative bone disease. False negative bone scans may be seen in cases of very aggressive tumours inducing little osteoblastic repair. It may also be seen in diffuse metastatic disease where radioisotope accumulation may be sufficiently uniform to produce a false-negative impression (superscans). Clues to the detection of the so-called superscan include skeletal uptake of greater-than-normal intensity, in relation to the background of the soft tissue and the low or absent uptake in the kidneys.

Q11. Answer B

DEXA stands for dual energy X-ray absorptiometry and is primarily used to study bone mineral density (BMD). A DEXA scan takes approximately 10–20 minutes to perform depending on the body parts being scanned. Two X-ray beams with differing energy levels are passed through specific bones such as the hip or the lower spine. BMD can be determined from the relative absorption of each beam and subtracting soft tissue absorption. A T-score can then be calculated by comparing the X-ray absorption on the study to reference values for a young healthy adult. WHO criteria defines osteoporosis as a BMD that lies 2.5 standard deviations below that of a healthy subject and this merits immediate initiation of corrective treatment. All men due to be commenced on androgen deprivation therapy (ADT) should have a baseline DEXA scan. During long-term ADT, it may be necessary to introduce regular measurements of BMD based on the initial T-score. BMD should be measured every 2 years if the initial T-score is above −1.0, or every year if the T-score is between −1.0 and −2.5, in the absence of associated risk factors. The risk of bony fractures in men receiving ADT for prostate cancer is 19.4% at 5 years and 40% at 15 years. Contra-indications to DEXA scanning include: Pregnancy and recent administration of a contrast agent, e.g., barium into the gastrointestinal tract.

References and Further Reading
Shahinian VB, Kuo YF, Freeman JL, and Goodwin JS. Risk of fracture after androgen deprivation for prostate cancer. *New England Journal of Medicine* (2005) 352: 154–164.

Q12. Answer D

Non-ionic contrast agents are 5–10 times safer that ionic agents. Ionic contrast agents such as Urografin have high osmolality (≥1200 mOsm/kg) and an allergy rate of 1/500. Non-ionic contrast agents such as Omnipaque have low osmolality (approximately 600 mOsm/kg) and an allergy rate of 1/2500. In patients with an eGFR > 60 mL/min Metformin does not have to be stopped if less than 100 mL of the contrast agent is being administered intravenously. If >100 mL is being administered or the eGFR is below 60 mL/min, Metformin should be withheld for 48 hours. There is a risk of developing nephrogenic systemic fibrosis (NSF) with the use of gadolinium-based contrast agents (GBCA) in patients with renal failure. NSF is a fibrosing disorder of skin and internal organs in patients with renal insufficiency exposed to GBCA during imaging studies (MRI). The onset of NSF symptoms usually occurs within days to months following exposure to GBCA in the vast majority of patients; however, in rare cases, symptoms have appeared years after the last reported exposure. Anaphylactoid hypersensitivity reactions to intravenous contrast agents are a medical emergency and should be managed as per the UK Resuscitation Council guidelines on emergency treatment of anaphylactic reactions. Specific treatment includes intramuscular administration of 0.5 mg (0.5 mL) of 1:1000 adrenaline, to be repeated after five minutes. This should be supplemented with an antihistamine agent such as chlorpheniramine 10 mg IV and hydrocortisone 200 mg IV.

References and Further Reading

Emergency treatment of anaphylactic reactions. Guidelines for healthcare providers. Working Group of the Resuscitation Council, London, UK, 2008.

Standards for intravascular contrast agent administration to adult patients, Third Edition. London, UK: The Royal College of Radiologists, 2015.

Q13. Answer A

The components of a cystoscope are the rod-lens telescope, a bridge, an obturator and an outer sheath. Telescopes are available with varying optical angles at their tips to aid different procedures within the urological tract. Telescopes are often colour-coded with bands around their light lead connector:

0° telescopes have green bands

30° telescopes have red bands

70° telescopes have yellow bands

The Hopkins Rod-Lens telescope consists of long tubes of glass separated by small lenses of air which improves light passage and overall vision. It is fibre optics which use the concept of total internal reflection for the passage of light or images down a fibre. Cystoscopes range between 17 and 25 French in external diameter.

References and Further Reading

Nakayama DK. How technology shaped modern surgery. *The American Surgeon* (2018) 84(6): 753–760.

EMQs – ANSWERS

Q14. Answer A

Q15. Answer G

Q16. Answer E

Q17. Answer F

Q18. Answer H

Q19. Answer B

The effects of ionising radiation on tissues depend on the radiation type and the tissue weighting. Energy absorption depends on the radiation energy and mass of tissue. It is measured in Gray (Gy), which is defined as the absorption of 1 Joule of energy in the form of ionising radiation, per 1 kg of matter. The equivalent dose on biological tissues is expressed in sievert (Sv). Diagnostic medical ultrasound waves operate at frequencies in the range of 2–18 MHz. Lower frequencies are used to study deeper tissues, as the attenuation of sound waves is greater at higher frequencies. A transrectal ultrasound probe for the assessment of the prostate gland employs a frequency of 7 MHz and the transabdominal ultrasound probes work best at a frequency around 3.5 MHz.

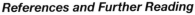

References and Further Reading
Mettler FA, Huda W, Yoshizumi TT, and Mahesh M. Effective doses in radiology and diagnostic nuclear medicine: A catalog. *Radiology* (2008) 248(1): 254–263.

Q20. Answer B

Q21. Answer C

Q22. Answer H

Q23. Answer F

Q24. Answer A

Q25. Answer I

The gold standard assessment for renal colic is a non-contrast CT KUB. In trauma any episode of frank haematuria needs a CT scan to assess the kidneys. In the mountain bike accident scenario, there is a possibility of a straddle injury; therefore, the bladder also needs to be assessed. EAU recommends a 10–15 minute follow-up CT scan after intravenous contrast in trauma imaging to check on the integrity of the collecting systems. Suspected testicular torsion cannot be ruled out with any form of imaging and therefore should always be surgically exploration urgently. In haemodynamically unstable patients, resuscitation and urgent surgical exploration in theatre is paramount, rather than arranging imaging investigations in the radiology department. Ideally an on-table IVU should be performed to check for the presence of a functioning contralateral kidney, if a trauma nephrectomy is being considered. It is usual practice to obtain a CT urogram to investigate the upper tracts in patients with visible haematuria. Patients with likely muscle invasive bladder cancer need full staging evaluation with a CT of the thorax, abdomen and pelvis to visualise metastatic disease to guide further treatment.

Q26. Answer C

Q27. Answer D

Q28. Answer B

Q29. Answer G

Q30. Answer H

Q31. Answer F

A major side effect of hormonal treatment for prostate cancer is osteoporosis. Osteoporosis leads to increased risk of fractures. All men being commenced on androgen deprivation therapy for the management of their prostate cancer should have a baseline DEXA scan with continued monitoring depending on their initial DEXA scan T-score. Spinal cord compression is another serious complication seen in some patients with prostate cancer. If suspected an MRI whole spine needs to be organised as a matter of urgency. Treatment options for spinal cord compression include surgery or radiotherapy; radiotherapy being more commonly practiced in the UK. Patients with localised prostate cancer need to be staged as per the recommendations in the EAU guidelines. The gentleman described in scenario 28 has high-risk, low-volume prostate cancer. With a presenting PSA greater than 20 and a Gleason score of 8he would need a staging bone scan as well as a multiparametric MRI of the prostate, to guide on suitability for radical treatment. Elderly patients may avoid the side effects of androgen depravation in asymptomatic locally advanced prostate cancer and so should be staged with a bone scan to ensure they do not have metastatic disease.

EAU guidelines recommend a multiparametric MRI in patients with negative prostate biopsies and a rising PSA to guide further biopsies. ^{11}C-Choline PET is more sensitive than CT or bone scan in identifying metastatic disease in patients with PSA less than 10 post radical treatment. This is likely to be superseded by PSMA PET in the future. PSMA (Prostate-specific membrane antigen) PET scan has been extensively studied, and different PSMA ligands have been used for this purpose including [68]gallium and [18]fluorine-labeled PET probes. PSMA PET imaging can be used to evaluate biochemical recurrence, even at low PSA levels. It has shown interesting applications for tumour detection, primary staging, assessment of therapeutic responses and treatment planning.

References and Further Reading

EAU – ESTRO – ESUR – SIOG Guidelines on Prostate Cancer. Mottet N, Bellmunt J, Briers E, Bolla M, Bourke L, Cornford P, De Santis M, Henry A, Joniau S, Lam T, Mason MD, Van den Poel H, Van den Kwast TH, Rouvière O, Wiegel T; members of the EAU – ESTRO – ESUR – SIOG Prostate Cancer Guidelines Panel. Edn. presented at the EAU Annual Congress London 2017. 978-90-79754-91-5. Publisher: EAU Guidelines Office. Place published: Arnhem, the Netherlands.

Q32. Answer B

Q33. Answer A

Q34. Answer C

Q35. Answer A

Q36. Answer B

Q37. Answer C

KTP green light laser has a wavelength of 532 nm, with a tissue penetration depth of 0.8 mm. It is used to perform a relatively bloodless vaporisation of BPH tissue. Nd:YAG has a wavelength of 1064 nm and a tissue penetration depth of 3–5 mm. It is most commonly used for incising strictures and treating superficial penile cancers. Ho:YAG or holmium laser has a wavelength of 2140 nm and a tissue penetration depth of 0.4 mm. It is safe to use in the ureter and is commonly employed for intracorporeal lithotripsy.

Q38. Answer A

Q39. Answer F

Q40. Answer G

A CT of the abdomen and pelvis without a contrast cystogram only detects 50% of bladder injuries. This can be improved to an almost 100% detection rate by the addition of a cystogram. Any patient with frank haematuria following trauma needs an accurate renal and bladder assessment. Ureteric injuries are also possible but rare.

Injury to the urethra is usually associated with severe pelvic trauma in males. Investigations for urethral trauma should be initiated in the presence of pelvic fractures, straddle injuries or penetrating trauma in the vicinity of the urethra and in penile fractures. A retrograde urethrogram should be performed and a delayed CT scan considered in such trauma patients. Catheterisation has been dismissed as a diagnostic tool as it can turn a partial urethral tear into a complete urethral disruption, increase haemorrhage and the risk of infection in sterile haematuria; however, if a functional urethral catheter is already in place, it should not be removed.

Q41. Answer B

Q42. Answer E

Q43. Answer D

Q44. Answer F

Gram staining helps differentiate bacteria into two categories based on the proportion of peptidoglycan in their cell walls. A thick cell wall in Gram-positive bacteria helps retain the purple crystal violet-iodine complex, whereas Gram-negative bacteria with a thinner peptidoglycan layer lose their purple colour during a washing process with alcohol or acetone. Application of a counterstain with safranin or basic carbol fuchsin gives the Gram-negative bacteria a pink or red colour. Ziehl–Neelsen (ZN) staining is used to detect acid-fast organisms and mainly mycobacteria, e.g., *Mycobacterium tuberculosis*. Mycobacteria have thick waxy lipid coats which are otherwise difficult to stain using ordinary methods such as the Gram stain. Acid-fast bacilli stain bright red with the ZN stain. Chlamydia is the most commonly reported bacterial sexually transmitted infection. The Nucleic Acid Amplification Test (NAAT) is a highly sensitive and commonly used investigation designed to detect the genetic material (DNA) of the chlamydia bacteria. A polymerase chain reaction (PCR) test is an example of a nucleic acid amplification test. Papanicolaou staining is most commonly used for the cytological assessment of exfoliated cells. It involves a multichromatic staining technique using five dyes in three solutions based on aqueous haematoxylin with multiple counterstaining dyes, giving great transparency and delicacy of detail. It is particularly useful in screening for cancer. Haematoxylin and eosin is most widely used histological stain. Cell nuclei stain blue with haematoxylin and counterstaining with eosin stains the cytoplasm in various shades of pink or red. Hale's colloidal iron stains the entire cytoplasm of chromophobe renal cell carcinoma cells blue and can thus usually be distinguished from oncocytoma, where only the cell border stains blue.

Q45. Answer B

Q46. Answer D

Q47. Answer C

Q48. Answer G

Diathermy or electrosurgery uses high frequency alternating current to generate localised heat which can be used to cut or coagulate tissues. Current is the rate at which electrons or ions flow along a conductive path/electric circuit. Voltage is the force that enables electrons or ions to move through a circuit or conductor. Resistance refers to heat being generated when electrons meet resistance to their flow. Overall power is measured in Watts and is the interaction between current, voltage, resistance and time Pure CUT has a continuous, high power, low voltage waveform. High current density heats tissues (up to 1000°C) quickly causing them to swell and explode resulting in a clean cutting incision. COAG has an intermittent, low-power, high-voltage waveform. Lower current density results in a slower heating effect, and high voltage produces sparks dissipating heat over a larger area. A Blend setting on the diathermy machine allows for the combined effect of COAG and CUT.

Q49. Answer E

Q50. Answer D

Q51. Answer D

Q52. **Answer E**

Contamination – Soiling or pollution of inanimate objects or living material with harmful, potentially infectious or undesirable substances. Decontamination – A process that removes or destroys contamination, so that infectious agents cannot reach a susceptible site in sufficient quantities. Cleaning – A process that physically removes infectious agents and the organic matter on which they thrive but not necessarily destroy them. Disinfection – A process that reduces the number of viable infectious agents but may not necessarily inactivate some microbial agents such as spores and certain viruses. Sterilisation – A validated process used to render a product free from viable microorganisms. A widely used method for sterilisation is using steam in an autoclave. The sterilisation time depends on the temperature applied: at 140°, it can be completed in four minutes. Other sterilisation methods include use of dry heat, gamma radiation, or ethylene oxide. The level of cleaning needed depends on whether the equipment is going to be in contact with the mucous membranes and whether it would result in a penetrating contact. Any breach of mucous membrane or skin requires the equipment to be sterilised. If the equipment only comes into contact with mucous membranes, without breaching them a process of disinfection is required. Examples of disinfectants include alcohol and aldehydes. Flexible cystoscopes require high-level disinfection. Various chemicals can be used for this purpose, including the germicide chlorine dioxide, Cidex and glutaradehyde.

Q53. **Answer F**

Q54. **Answer B**

Q55. **Answer D**

Q56. **Answer E**

The French gauge corresponds to three times the diameter in mm. Adult cystoscopes range from 17 to 25 Fr. A 21 Fr cystoscope has an external diameter of 7 mm. Resectoscopes range from 26 to 28 Fr. Semi-rigid ureteroscopes can range from 7 to 10 Fr at their tip. Flexible ureteroscopes can range from 5 to 9 Fr at their tip, depending on the manufacturer. The working channels of flexible ureteroscopes are usually in the order of 3 to 4 Fr, depending on the bore of the ureteroscope. Guide wires are generally 0.035–0.038 inches in diameter, and baskets can vary from 1.3 to 3 Fr.

CHAPTER 6: PROSTATE CANCER

Simon R. J. Bott and Amr Emara

MCQs

Q1. Which of the following is TRUE regarding adenocarcinoma of the prostate?
- A. Is the fourth commonest cause of male cancer death in the UK.
- B. Is more common in men than breast carcinoma is in women.
- C. Is more common in the transition zone than in the peripheral zone.
- D. Has never been recorded in patients with congenital 5α-reductase deficiency.
- E. The critical feature in the pathological diagnosis is preservation of basal cell layer.

Q2. Which of the following is NOT a recognised side effect of LHRH agonists in the treatment of carcinoma of the prostate?
- A. Osteoporosis
- B. An initial drop in plasma testosterone
- C. Gynaecomastia
- D. Hot flushes
- E. Erectile dysfunction

Q3. Which of the following is TRUE regarding brachytherapy monotherapy for prostate cancer?
- A. Should be considered in the management of intermediate- and high-risk localised prostate cancer.
- B. HDR uses palladium[103] as the radioactive source.
- C. Low dose rate (permanent seed implantation) (LDR) and high dose rate (HDR) temporary implantation represent the two types of brachytherapy.
- D. There is no limitation in relation to prostate size.

- E. A 'PSA bounce' is less common after brachytherapy than after external beam radiotherapy.

Q4. Which finding is TRUE in the Scandinavian Prostate Cancer Group Study Number 4 (SPCG-4), comparing radical prostatectomy versus watchful waiting in the management of early prostate cancer after up to 10 years follow-up?
- A. Radical prostatectomy reduces prostate cancer-specific mortality, overall mortality, the risks of metastasis and local progression compared with watchful waiting.
- B. Radical prostatectomy has no benefit in terms of overall survival.
- C. Radical prostatectomy has no benefit in terms of disease specific survival.
- D. Radical prostatectomy has no benefit in terms of reducing prostate cancer-specific mortality, overall mortality, the risks of metastasis or local progression.
- E. With longer follow up any difference in terms of cancer specific survival between the radical prostatectomy and watchful waiting is likely to decrease.

Q5. Which of the following drugs have shown efficacy in the treatment of 'hot flushes' following hormonal treatment for advanced prostate cancer?
- A. Diethylstilbestrol
- B. 5α-reductase inhibitors
- C. Medroxyprogesterone acetate
- D. Tamsulosin
- E. Clonidine

Q6. In the report of the American Joint Committee on Cancer (2018), which of the following is CORRECT?
   A. T1c disease may be visible using multi-parametric MRI.
   B. Non-regional lymph node involvement is defined as N2.
   C. Tumour invading into, but not through, the capsule is defined as pT3a disease.
   D. pT3b indicates involvement of the seminal vesicles after radical prostatectomy.
   E. Impalpable prostate cancer present in both lobes in TRUS biopsies is defined as T1b.

Q7. Which of the following is TRUE regarding the pathogenesis of prostate cancer?
   A. If 2 or more first-degree relatives have prostate cancer the risk of developing the disease increases 5–11 fold.
   B. It is estimated 20% are hereditary.
   C. Japanese men have a lower incidence of latent/indolent disease than US men.
   D. In the US, African American men have a lower incidence and mortality from prostate cancer than White American men.
   E. Increasing age is not a risk factor for developing prostate cancer.

Q8. In the Prostate Cancer Prevention Trial, how many men over 62 years old with a normal PSA (≤4 ng/mL) and a normal rectal examination had prostate cancer on TRUS biopsy and how many men with cancer had Gleason ≥7 disease?
   A. 5% and 2.5%
   B. 8% and 2%
   C. 10% and 5%
   D. 15% and 15%
   E. 30% and 10%

Q9. Which of the following is CORRECT regarding men with localised prostate cancer treated with radiotherapy?
   A. Dose escalation from 70–80 Gy does not affect biochemical survival at 5 years.
   B. Prophylactic lymph node irradiation improves cancer specific survival in high-risk patients.
   C. There is no subsequent increased risk of developing bladder cancer.
   D. Recurrence is defined as a rise in PSA of >1 ng/mL above a PSA nadir.
   E. In men with Gleason 8–10 disease the use of neoadjuvant and 2 years adjuvant androgen deprivation therapy has a significant effect on 10-year overall mortality.

Q10. Which of the following information on molecular markers in prostate cancer is CORRECT?
   A. PCA3, a non-coding RNA, is under expressed in prostate cancer.
   B. Ki-67 antigen is detected by immunohistochemical staining and correlates with outcome after radical prostatectomy.
   C. Kallikrein 3 level is reduced in metastatic prostate cancer.
   D. High molecular weight cytokeratin binds to prostate cancer cells confirming the diagnosis of cancer over HGPIN.
   E. PSA doubling time is a useful tool that outperforms total PSA in the diagnosis of prostate cancer.

EMQs

Q11–14. Management of prostate cancer patients after radical treatment
   A. Hormonal therapy is routinely recommended.
   B. Biopsy of the prostate should be performed.
   C. Treatment should be offered when the PSA is <0.5 ng/mL.
   D. Docetaxel should be offered after checking eGFR.
   E. Abiraterone is first line treatment.
   F. Salvage brachytherapy should be offered.
   G. An isotope bone scan should be performed.

Choose the most appropriate management steps in the following situations:

Q11. In men with lymph node involvement in the pathology specimen after radical prostatectomy.

Q12. Patient considered for salvage radiotherapy after biochemical relapse post radical prostatectomy.

Q13. Biochemical relapse post radical radiotherapy in men considered for local salvage therapy.

Q14. In the investigation of patients with high-grade prostate cancer treated with radiotherapy with a post-treatment PSA doubling time of less than 3 months.

Q15–18. Hormonal treatment for prostate cancer
  A. Degarelix
  B. Bicalutamide
  C. Leuprolide
  D. Oestrogen
  E. Abiraterone
  F. Cyproterone acetate
  G. Surgical castration
  H. Enzalutamide

For each of the modes of action below, please match the hormonal treatment above.

Q15. Act by inhibiting CYP17 (17α-hydroxylase/C17,20-lyase)

Q16. Competitively inhibits the action of androgens by binding to cytosol androgen receptors in the target tissue

Q17. Binds reversibly to the pituitary GnRH receptors

Q18. Down regulation of pituitary GnRH receptors

Q19–20. PSA cut-off markers
  A. >0.18
  B. <0.75
  C. <0.15
  D. <0.35
  E. <0.01
  F. <0.18
  G. >0.25
  H. >0.35

For each of the PSA derivatives below, match the cut-off best defining a low likelihood of significant prostate cancer.

Q19. PSA density

Q20. Free to total PSA

Q21–23. Treatment options for patients with prostate cancer and a 10-year life expectancy
  A. Active surveillance, radical prostatectomy, brachytherapy and external beam radiotherapy
  B. Radical prostatectomy, brachytherapy, external beam radiotherapy
  C. Radical prostatectomy +/– adjuvant radiotherapy or external beam radiotherapy and hormonal manipulation
  D. Watchful waiting
  E. Focal therapy for prostate cancer in a trial setting

For each of the following scenarios, which of the above treatment options would be the best choice?

Q21. PSA is 6.2 ng/mL with Gleason score 4 + 4 (group 4) disease in 4 cores from a targeted biopsy, random biopsies are all negative, and the MRI scan demonstrates probable T3a disease

Q22. PSA is 4.7 ng/mL and Gleason 3 + 3 (group 1) disease in 1 of 24 cores taken, MRI PIRAD 3 – diffuse low signal in cores and clinical T1c disease

Q23. PSA is 7.2, an MRI shows a 6mm Gleason 3 + 4 = 7 (group 2) disease in a discrete area in a patient wanting treatment but wishing to minimise the risk of bowel, bladder and erectile dysfunction

Q24–27. Contemporary publications in prostate cancer
  A. There was no significant reduction in all-cause or prostate-cancer mortality between the two groups.
  B. Increased risk of death from prostate cancer or prostate cancer related treatment.

C. Prostate cancer mortality was reduced by 21%.

D. Prostate cancer mortality was reduced by almost a half.

E. Prostate cancer mortality was reduced by almost a third.

For the following clinical studies, choose the best conclusion from the list above.

Q24. The Prostate Cancer Intervention versus Observation Trial (PIVOT) comparing radical prostatectomy and observation

Q25. The European Randomised Study of Screening for Prostate Cancer (ERSPC)

Q26. Prostate, Lung, Colorectal and Ovarian (PLCO) Cancer Screening Trial

Q27. The Göteborg (became Swedish arm of ERSPC) randomised population-based prostate-cancer screening trial

Q28–30. Multi-parametric MR imaging (mp-MRI) of the prostate

A. On T2 imaging a circumscribed, homogenous moderately hypointense focus or mass ≥1.5 cm in greatest dimension or definite extraprostatic extension

B. On T2 imaging in the transition zone a lenticular or non-circumscribed, homogenous moderately hypointense, and <1.5 cm in greatest dimension

C. On T2-weighted imaging a wedge-shaped area of hypointensity and indistinct hypointense on ADC

D. Looking at Dynamic Contrast Enhanced (DCE) sequences focal and earlier than or contemporaneously with enhancement of adjacent normal prostatic tissues, and corresponding to suspicious finding on T2 and/or DWI

E. No early enhancement after contrast administration, or diffuse enhancement not corresponding to a focal finding on T2W and/or DWI or focal enhancement corresponding to a lesion demonstrating features of benign prostatic hyperplasia on T2W

For each of the following scenarios, which of the above imaging options would be the best choice?

Q28. Positive on DCE

Q29. A PI-RAD 5 lesion (significant tumour highly likely)

Q30. A PI-RAD 2 lesion (significant tumour unlikely)

MCQs – ANSWERS

Q1. Answer D

Prostate cancer is the second leading cause of male cancer death in the UK. The incidence of breast cancer exceeds that of prostate cancer in the UK (55,200 vs. 47,740, respectively). In total, about 75% of adenocarcinoma arise from the peripheral zone with the rest arising from the transition zone. Neither benign prostate hyperplasia (BPH) nor prostate cancer has ever been reported in patients with 5α-reductase deficiency. Absence of the basal layer distinguishes malignant from benign prostate acini.

Q2. Answer B

The plasma testosterone initially rises (the tumour flare), so an anti-androgen, such as bicalutamide, is given for 3 days before and 3 weeks after starting an LHRH agonist. The remainder all are recorded side effects for androgen deprivation therapy, anti-androgens have similar side effects but with better preservation of potency and libido.

Q3. Answer C

According to NICE guidelines brachytherapy is considered an option in low- and intermediate-risk groups. Iridium[192] is the radioisotope used in high dose brachytherapy in combination with external beam radiotherapy. Iodine[125] and palladium[103] are used in low dose brachytherapy. Prostate volume of 50–60 mL is considered the upper limit for BXT treatment due to pubic arch interference preventing insertion of the source in some of the anterior gland.

Further Reading

Georgios Koukourakis et al. Brachytherapy for Prostate Cancer: A Systematic Review, Advances in *Urology*, Volume 2009, Article ID 327945, 11 pages.

Q4. Answer A

Radical prostatectomy reduces disease-specific mortality, overall mortality and the risks of metastasis and local progression compared with watchful waiting after up to 10 years follow-up.

Further Reading

Bill-Axelson A, Radical prostatectomy or watchful waiting in prostate cancer–29-Year follow-up. *N Eng J Med* 2018; 379: 2319–2329.

Q5. Answer C

Medroxyprogesterone 20 mg od has been shown to significantly reduce hot flushes; cyproterone acetate also reduces flushes.

Further Reading

Irani J et al. Efficacy of venlafaxine, medroxyprogesterone acetate, and cyproterone acetate for the treatment of vasomotor hot flushes in men taking gonadotropin-releasing hormone analogues for prostate cancer: A double-blind, randomised trial. *Lancet Oncol* 2010; 11(2): 147–154.

Q6. Answer D

T1 disease is not palpable or visible with imaging, non-regional (extrapelvic) lymph node involvement is classified M1a. Tumour involving but not penetrating through the capsule is pT2 (p denotes 'pathological'). Tumour found in both lobes by needle biopsy, but not palpable or visible by imaging, is classified as T1c.

Q7. Answer A

It is estimated 9% of prostate cancer is hereditary, other risk factors include ethnicity and increasing age, the incidence of latent/indolent prostate cancer is very similar throughout the world.

Q8. Answer D

The 'Prostate Cancer Prevention Trial' (PCPT) randomised 18,882 men to either finasteride or placebo. Eligibility criteria were prostate specific antigen (PSA) <3 ng/mL, age ≥55 years and a normal digital rectal examination (DRE). Participants underwent yearly PSA and DRE checks. A 6-core biopsy was performed if the PSA rose to 4 ng/mL. Overall a 25% relative risk and 4% absolute reduction in prostate cancer was seen, primarily tumours ≤Gleason 6. However, an absolute 15% increase in Gleason 7 and above tumours was seen in the treatment arm.

Further Reading

Thompson IM, Pauler DK, Goodman PJ, et al. Prevalence of prostate cancer among men with a prostate-specific antigen level ≤4.0 ng per milliliter. *N Engl J Med* 2004; 350(22): 2239–2246.

Thompson IM et al. The influence of finasteride on the development of prostate cancer. *N Engl J Med* 2003; 349(3): 215–224.

Thompson IM et al. Effect of finasteride on the sensitivity of PSA for detecting prostate cancer. *J Natl Cancer Inst* 2006; 98(16): 1128–1133.

Thompson IM, Jr. et al. Long-term survival of participants in the prostate cancer prevention trial. *N Engl J Med* 2013; 369(7): 603–610.

Q9. Answer E

The RTOG 9292 study reported significant improvement in local control, the development of metastases and disease-free survival in patients receiving long-term ADT and overall survival in men with GS 8–10 disease. Numerous studies demonstrate the benefit of dose escalation, there is no good evidence that pelvic irradiation is of benefit in N0 disease. Radiotherapy does increase the risk of bladder cancer by 2.3x and rectal cancer by 1.7x. The Phoenix Consensus Conference definition of PSA failure (with an accuracy of >80% for clinical failure) is any PSA increase >2 ng/mL higher than the PSA nadir value, regardless of the serum concentration of the nadir.

Q10. Answer B

PCA3 is overexpressed in prostate cancer, kallikrein 3 is also known as PSA so rises in metastatic disease, high molecular weight cytokeratin binds basal cells – malignant acini lack basal cells. PSA doubling time and PSA velocity provide limited predictive information over PSA alone in prostate cancer diagnosis.

EMQs – ANSWERS

Q11. Answer A

Q12. Answer C

Q13. Answer B

Q14. Answer G

The Messing study demonstrated improved survival in men with N1 disease at Radical Prostatectomy receiving androgen deprivation vs. placebo. Patients considered for salvage therapy post radiotherapy should normally have a biopsy of the prostate to confirm local recurrence, as well as pelvic MRI. Patients should be offered salvage radiotherapy post radical prostatectomy while the PSA is still low (i.e., up to 0.5 µmol/L), to improve cancer outcome.

Q15. Answer E

Q16. Answer B

Q17. Answer A

Q18. Answer C

Prostate cancer is influenced by androgens, 90% of which are secreted by the testes and 10% by the adrenal glands. The hypothalamic-pituitary-gonadal axis controls their secretion. Luteinising hormone-releasing hormone (LHRH) from the hypothalamus stimulates the anterior pituitary to secrete luteinizing hormone (LH), which stimulates the Leydig cells of the testes to secrete testosterone. LHRH antagonists/agonists or bilateral orchidectomy disrupt the hypothalamic-pituitary-gonadal axis. Abiraterone is a CYP17 inhibitor which prevents intra-cellular testosterone synthesis and is usually administered alongside prednisolone. Enzalutamide is an anti-androgen that blocks the androgen receptor and also prevents its translocation and transcription.

Q19. Answer C

Q20. Answer G

The PSA density (PSAD) is calculated by dividing the serum PSA value by the prostate volume in mL. The most commonly used cut off for a reassuring PSAD is <0.15 ng/mL^2. PSA is a proteolytic enzyme so most is bound in plasma to alpha 1-antichymotrypsin, some is unbound (free) and a very small fraction of PSA is bound to other protease inhibitors (not measured by most lab assays). Higher total PSA levels and lower percentages of free PSA are associated with higher risks of prostate cancer When the total PSA is in the range of 4.0–10.0 ng/mL, a free:total PSA ratio ≤0.10 indicates 49% risk of prostate cancer; a free:total PSA ratio >0.25 indicates a 8% risk of prostate cancer. The cut-off of >0.25 is therefore the usual cut-off indicating a low risk of significant prostate cancer.

Q21. Answer C

Q22. Answer A

Q23. Answer E

NICE (2019) recommend active surveillance, radical prostatectomy or radical radiotherapy for men with low-risk localised prostate cancer and radical prostatectomy and radiotherapy for intermediate- and high-risk localised disease. Focal therapy (HIFU or cryosurgery) may be offered if part of a clinical trial comparing it with radical treatment options.

Q24. Answer A

Q25. Answer C

Q26. Answer A

Q27. Answer D

In both the US PIVOT trial, which compared radical prostatectomy and observation with follow-up nearly 20 years, and the PLCO US PSA screening trial, there was no significant reduction in all-cause or prostate-cancer mortality between the intervention versus control groups. The ERSPC PSA screening trial showed after a median follow-up of 11 years, the risk of death from prostate cancer in the screening group was 21% and 29% after adjusting for noncompliance. After the most recent update, the NNS was 570 and NND was 18 (previously was 26). The Göteborg screening study showed a 40% reduction in mortality in the screened group after 14 years of follow-up. The larger reduction seen in the study was due to lack of contamination in the control arm, more frequent testing (every 2 years) and starting PSA testing at a younger age (50 years).

Further Reading

Wilt T. Follow-up of prostatectomy versus observation for early prostate cancer. *N Engl J Med* 2017; 377: 132–142.

Schröder FH et al. Prostate-cancer mortality at 11 years of follow-up. *N Engl J Med* 2012; 366(11): 981–990.

Schröder FH et al. Screening and prostate cancer mortality: Results of the European Randomised study of screening for prostate cancer (ERSPC) at 13 years of follow-up. *Lancet.* 2014; 384(9959): 2027–2035.

Andriole GL. Mortality results from a randomized prostate-cancer screening trial. *N Engl J Med* 2009; 360(13): 1310.

Hugosson J et al. Mortality results from the Göteborg randomised prostate cancer screening trial. *Lancet Oncol* 2010; 11(8): 725–732.

Q28. Answer D

Q29. Answer A

Q30. Answer C

The PI-RADS (Prostate Imaging Reporting and Data System) refers to a structured reporting protocol for evaluating the prostate for prostate cancer prior to treatment. The score is calculated based on T2-weighted images, a dynamic contrast study (DCE) and diffusion-weighted imaging (DWI).

A score is given according to each variable. The scale is based on a score from 1 to 5 (which is given for each lesion), with 1 being highly likely benign and 5 being highly suspicious of malignancy.

Further Reading

Mundy AR, Fitzpatrick J, Neal DE, George NJ. *The Scientific Basis of Urology.* Third Edition. London: CRC Press, 2010.

Bott S, Patel U, Djavan B, Carroll PR. *Images in Urology.* London: Springer, 2012.

CHAPTER 7: BLADDER CANCER

Vineet Agrawal, Lyndon Gommersall and David Mak

MCQs

Q1. Regarding bladder cancer, the following statements are true EXCEPT?
 A. The estimated male:female ratio is 2:1.
 B. At the initial diagnosis of bladder cancer, 75% of cases are diagnosed as non-muscle-invasive bladder cancer and approximately 25% as muscle-invasive disease.
 C. Approximately one-third of patients diagnosed with muscle-invasive disease have undetected metastasis at the time of treatment of the primary tumour.
 D. 25% of patients subjected to radical cystectomy present with lymph node involvement at the time of surgery.

Q2. Tobacco smoking is the most well-established risk factor for bladder cancer, causing 50%–65% of male cases and 20%–30% of female cases. Which of the following statements regarding smoking and bladder cancer is TRUE?
 A. A causal relationship has not been established between an exposure to tobacco and cancer in studies in which chance, bias and confounding factors can be ruled out with reasonable confidence.
 B. A meta-analysis reporting on pooled risk estimates for current and former smokers demonstrated a significant association with bladder cancer for current smokers only.
 C. There is no immediate decrease in the risk of bladder cancer in those who stop smoking.

 D. The promotion of smoking cessation would result in the incidence of bladder cancer decreasing equally in men and women.

Q3. A 69-year-old male has undergone a radical cysto-prostatectomy for muscle-invasive bladder cancer with no histo-logical evidence of peri-vesical invasion. Staging investigations included a CT of the chest and abdomen, which showed no metastasis. However, histology of the lymphadenectomy specimen showed that two lymph nodes in the external iliac group were positive for metastasis. What would be the correct TNM (2017) pathological staging?
 A. pT2 pN1 M0
 B. pT3 pN1 M0
 C. pT2 pN2 M0
 D. pT2 pN3 M0

Q4. Regarding the molecular biology of bladder cancer pathogenesis, the following are true, EXCEPT:
 A. Chromosome 10 loss of heterozygosity (LOH) is found in more than 50% of all bladder tumours.
 B. Low-grade pTa tumours usually have alterations in the RAS-MAP kinase signal transduction pathway, the most frequent being fibroblast growth factor receptor 3 (FGFR3) mutations on chromosome 4p.
 C. Over-expression of the genes that encode receptor tyrosine kinases such as EGFR (epidermal growth

factor receptor) and the Erb2 receptor have been reported.

D. Muscle-invasive tumours and CIS frequently have alterations in the p53 and retinoblastoma (pRb) pathways that control the cell cycle.

Q5. Which of the following statements is FALSE regarding fluorescence-guided biopsy or photodynamic diagnosis (PDD) and resection?

A. The value of fluorescence cystoscopy for improvement of the outcome in relation to progression rate or survival has not been proven.

B. The additional detection rate with PDD for all tumours is about 35% and about 40% for CIS.

C. False positivity can occur due to recent TUR and during the first three months after BCG instillation.

D. A large, multicentre, RCT comparing hexa-aminolaevulinic acid (HAL) fluorescence guided TUR with standard TUR reported an absolute reduction of no more than 9% in the recurrence rate within 9 months in the HAL arm.

Q6. Regarding non-muscle-invasive bladder cancer and adjuvant chemo/immunotherapy, which of the following statement is FALSE?

A. Recent evidence suggests no statistically significant benefit from early postoperative chemotherapeutic instillation in patients with large or recurrent tumours (i.e., intermediate risk) or in those with high-risk NMIBC.

B. An EORTC meta-analysis showed that a single, immediate instillation of intravesical chemotherapy after TURBT results in a 11.7% absolute reduction in tumour recurrence (a decrease of 24% in the odds of recurrence). No significant differences in efficacy were noted among the chemotherapeutic agents studied, indicating that the choice of chemotherapeutic drug is optional.

C. An EORTC meta-analysis showed that compared to TURBT alone, immediate

adjuvant chemotherapy after TURBT significantly improves disease-free survival and reduces progression rates.

Q7. Intravesical immunotherapy results in a massive local immune response characterised by induced expression of cytokines in the urine and bladder wall and by an influx of granulocytes, mononuclear and dendritic cells. Which of the following statements regarding intravesical BCG immunotherapy is FALSE?

A. The mechanism of action includes direct binding of BCG to fibronectin within the bladder wall, subsequently leading to direct stimulation of cell-based immunologic response and an anti-angiogenic state.

B. Overall, response to intravesical immunotherapy may be limited if a patient has an immunosuppressive disease or by advanced age.

C. The original regimen described by Morales included an intramuscular dose, which was discontinued after success using a similar intravesical regimen.

D. The vaccine is reconstituted with 50 mL of saline and should be administered through a urethral catheter under gravity drainage soon thereafter to avoid aggregation.

Q8. The limits of dissection of a standard pelvic lymphadenectomy in cases of radical cystectomy include the following, EXCEPT:

A. Obturator nerve laterally

B. Bladder medially

C. Bifurcation of the common iliac artery cephalad

D. Endopelvic fascia caudally

Q9. A 69-year-old woman has been diagnosed with muscle-invasive bladder cancer and is considering undergoing radical cystectomy with formation of an orthotopic neobladder. Her GFR is 52 mL/min and she has marked right-sided hydronephrosis. Which of the following statements is TRUE?

A. She should be counselled that orthotopic neobladder is contraindicated in her case in view of the low GFR and presence of hydronephrosis.

B. Quality of life studies of patients with orthotopic diversion have uniformly shown that patients with continent diversions have a better quality of life than those with ileal conduits.

C. Her pre-operative counselling can be facilitated by results of several randomised controlled studies which have become available in the past few years comparing neobladder to ileal conduit and other types of urinary diversion.

D. If she had pre-existing significant stress incontinence, this would be a relative contra-indication for neobladder formation.

Q10. Which of the following statements regarding the use of bowel for urinary diversion is TRUE?

A. Mild metabolic acidosis may be expected in up to half of the patients after ileal conduit diversion.

B. The terminal ileum is the sole site of vitamin B12 and of bile acid absorption.

C. Normal serum pH and bicarbonate exclude a severely compensated metabolic acidosis.

D. The morbidity of radical cystectomy and urinary diversion is up to 25% diversion related.

EMQs

Q11–13. **Benign tumours of the bladder**
  A. Nephrogenic adenoma
  B. Epithelial metaplasia
  C. Leukoplakia
  D. Inverted papilloma
  E. Leiomyoma
  F. Cystitis cystica
  G. Cystitis glandularis
  H. Papilloma

For each of the following descriptions, select the most appropriate diagnosis from the list above. Each option may be used once, more than once or not at all.

Q11. Approximately, 40% of women and 5% of men have this condition, which is usually related to infection, trauma and surgery. Treatment is unnecessary.

Q12. Occasionally, present with coexistent urothelial cancer elsewhere in the urinary system, occurring more commonly in the upper tract than the bladder.

Q13. Previously been categorised as grade 1 Ta tumours of the bladder until the World Health Organization (WHO) changed the classification of non-invasive bladder cancer in 1998.

Q14–16. **Non-urothelial malignances**
  A. Sarcoma
  B. Small-cell carcinoma
  C. Squamous cell cancer
  D. Adenocarcinoma
  E. Signet ring cell carcinoma

For each of the following descriptions, select the most appropriate diagnosis from the list above. Each option may be used once, more than once or not at all.

Q14. In the majority of cases there are regional or distant metastases at the time of presentation, and the mean survival time is less than 20 months.

Q15. Tumour that is very sensitive to chemotherapy and the primary mode of treatment is usually chemo radiation therapy.

Q16. Chronic infection with *Schistosoma haematobium* leads to this type of bladder malignancy.

Q17–19. Urinary molecular markers tests for bladder cancer
  A. Bladder tumour antigen (BTA)
  B. Microsatellite analysis
  C. UroVysion
  D. ImmunoCyt
  E. Survivin
  F. Gene microarray
  G. Nuclear matrix protein 22 (NMP22)
  H. Cytokeratins

For each of the following descriptions, select the most appropriate test from the list above. Each option may be used once, more than once or not at all.

Q17. Point of care test, with higher sensitivity than urine cytology. Potentially can be used during follow up surveillance for bladder cancer.

Q18. Highest sensitivity for detection of low-grade tumours (60%) and is less affected by other urological diseases than other markers.

Q19. Utilises fluorescence in situ hybridisation (FISH).

Q20–22. Research trials in bladder cancer
  A. BOXIT
  B. HYMN
  C. ODMIT-C

For each of the following descriptions, select the most appropriate trial from the list above. Each option may be used once, more than once or not at all.

Q20. The only chemo-prevention trial in bladder cancer.

Q21. Addition of oral COX-2 inhibitors Celecoxib to standard therapy is more effective in terms of disease recurrence at three years compared with standard therapy alone for the treatment of non-muscle-invasive TCC of the bladder in intermediate- or high-risk groups.

Q22. A trial comparing hyperthermia and mitomycin chemotherapy with a second BCG treatment, or other standard treatment, for patients with recurrence of non-muscle-invasive bladder cancer following induction or maintenance BCG therapy.

Q23–25. Staging for upper urinary tract-urothelial cell carcinoma
  A. T1N0M0
  B. T1N1M0
  C. T2N1M0
  D. T2N2M0
  E. T3N1M0
  F. T3N2M0
  G. T4N1M0
  H. T4N2M0

Choose the most appropriate TNM staging according to the latest (2017) classification for upper urinary tract-urothelial cell carcinoma (UUT-UCC) from the list above. Each option may be used once, more than once or not at all.

Q23. Tumour invading muscle, metastasis in a single lymph node 1.5 cm, and no distant metastasis.

Q24. Tumour invades subepithelial connective tissue, no regional lymph node metastasis, and no distant metastasis.

Q25. Tumour invades beyond muscularis renal parenchyma, metastasis in two lymph nodes 2 cm each, no distant metastasis.

MCQs – ANSWERS

Q1. Answer A

The estimated male: female ratio for bladder cancer incidence is 3.8:1. However, women are more likely to be diagnosed with primary muscle-invasive disease than men. In a series of patients undergoing radical cystectomy for de novo muscle-invasive TCC, women were more likely to be diagnosed with muscle invasion primarily than men (85.2% and 50.7% respectively), probably as a lot of these women present with UTI's or irritative LUTS and are treated as such. Women are also more likely to be older than men when diagnosed, with a direct effect on their survival. In addition, delayed diagnosis is more likely in women after haematuria is observed because the differential diagnosis in women includes diseases more prevalent than bladder cancer.

The incidence rate of bladder cancer is highest in developed countries. 63% of all bladder cancer cases occur in developed countries with 55% from North America and Europe. There is a geographic difference in bladder cancer incidence rates across the world with the highest in Southern and Eastern Europe, parts of Africa, Middle East and North America and the lowest in Asia and underdeveloped areas in Africa. The incidence peaks in the seventh decade of life.

Superficial bladder cancer is much more common than muscle-invasive bladder cancer. However, among patients treated with radical cystectomy because of muscle-invasive disease, 57% had muscle invasion at presentation, while 43% had been initially diagnosed with non-muscle-invasive disease that progressed despite organ-preserving treatment.

Further Reading

1. Ploeg M, Aben KK, Kiemeney LA. The present and future burden of urinary bladder cancer in the world. *World J Urol* 2009; 27: 289–229.
2. Vaidya A, Soloway MS, Hawke C, et al. De novo muscle-invasive bladder cancer: Is there a change in trend? *J Urol* 2001; 165(1): 47–50.

Q2. Answer D

Smoking is responsible for 30%–50% of all bladder cancers in males, and smokers have a 2- to 6-fold greater risk of getting bladder cancer. A causal relationship has been established between an exposure to tobacco and cancer in studies in which chance, bias and confounding can be ruled out with reasonable confidence. A meta-analysis looked at 216 observational studies on cigarette smoking and cancer from 1961 to 2003, with reported estimates for current and/or former smokers. The pooled risk estimates for bladder cancer demonstrated a significant association for both current and former smokers. In an analysis of 21 studies, the overall relative risk calculated for current smokers was 2.77, while an analysis of 15 studies showed that the overall relative risk calculated for former smokers was 1.72.

Smoking cessation will decrease the risk of eventual urothelial cancer formation in a linear fashion. After 15 years of not smoking, the risk of cancer formation is the same as for a person who never smoked. The strong influence of smoking in bladder cancer formation prevents accurate determination of other less significant dietary, micronutrient, or lifestyle changes that may alter bladder cancer formation.

An immediate decrease in the risk of bladder cancer is observed in those who stopped smoking. The reduction was about 40% within 1–4 years of quitting smoking.

Further Reading

1. Vineis P, Kogevinas M, Simonato L, Brennan P, Boffetta P. Levelling-off of the risk of lung and bladder cancer in heavy smokers: An analysis based on multicentric case-control studies and a metabolic interpretation. *Mutat Res* 2000; 463(1): 103–110.

2. Boffetta P. Tobacco smoking and risk of bladder cancer. *Scand J Urol Nephrol Suppl* 2008; 42(218): 45–54. doi:10.1080/03008880802283664.

3. IARC Working Group on the Evaluation of Carcinogenic Risks to Humans. Tobacco smoke and involuntary smoking. *IARC Monogr Eval Carcinog Risks Hum* 2004; 83: 1–1438.

4. Gandini S, Botteri E, Iodice S, et al. Tobacco smoking and cancer: A meta-analysis. *Int J Cancer* 2008; 122(1): 155–164.

5. Brennan P, Bogillot O, Cordier S, et al. Cigarette smoking and bladder cancer in men: A pooled analysis of 11 case-control studies. *Int J Cancer* 2000; 86(2): 289–294.

Q3. Answer C

The Tumour, Node, Metastasis (TNM) Classification of Malignant Tumours is the method most widely used to classify the extent of cancer spread. An eighth edition was published in 2017.

2017 TNM Classification of Urinary Bladder Cancer

T – Primary tumour		
Tx	Primary tumour cannot be assessed	
T0	No evidence of primary tumour	
Ta	Non-invasive papillary carcinoma	
Tis	Carcinoma in situ: 'flat tumour'	
T1	Tumour invades subepithelial connective tissue	
T2	Tumour invades muscle	
	T2a	Tumour invades superficial muscle (inner half)
	T2b	Tumour invades deep muscle (outer half)
T3	Tumour invades perivesical tissue	
	T3a	Microscopically
	T3b	Macroscopically (extravesical mass)
T4	Tumour invades any of the following: prostate, uterus, vagina, pelvic wall, abdominal wall	
	T4a	Tumour invades prostate stroma, seminal vesicles, uterus or vagina
	T4b	Tumour invades pelvic wall or abdominal wall
N – Lymph nodes		
Nx	Regional lymph nodes cannot be assessed	
N0	No regional lymph node metastasis	
N1	Metastasis in a single lymph node in the true pelvis (hypogastric, obturator, external iliac or presacral)	
N2	Metastasis in multiple lymph nodes in the true pelvis (hypogastric, obturator, external iliac or presacral)	
N3	Metastasis in common iliac lymph node(s)	

M – Distant metastasis

> M0 No distant metastasis
>
> M1 Distant metastasis

WHO grading in 1973 and 2004

> 1973 WHO grading (widely used as most trials pertaining to bladder cancer used this)
>
> - Urothelial papilloma
> - Grade 1/2/3 – Well/ moderately/poorly differentiated

> 2004 WHO grading
>
> - Urothelial papilloma
> - Papillary urothelial neoplasm of low malignant potential (PUNLMP)
> - Low-grade papillary urothelial carcinoma
> - High-grade papillary urothelial carcinoma

Both CT and MR imaging may be used for assessment of local invasion, but they are unable to detect microscopic invasion of perivesical fat (T3a). The aim of CT and MR imaging is therefore to detect T3b disease or higher. The assessment of nodal status based simply on size is limited by the inability of both CT and MR imaging to identify metastases in normal sized or minimally enlarged nodes. Pelvic nodes greater than 8 mm and abdominal nodes greater than 10 mm in maximum short axis diameter should be regarded as enlarged on CT and MR imaging.

Sensitivities for detection of lymph node metastases are low, ranging from 48% to 87%. Specificities are also low as nodal enlargement may be due to benign pathology.

The pN (pathological Node) category is closely related to the number of lymph nodes studied by the pathologist. For this reason, some authors have observed that more than nine lymph nodes have to be investigated to reflect pN0 appropriately after cystectomy.

Further Reading

1. EAU Guidelines on Bladder Cancer Muscle-invasive and Metastatic. Chairman A. Stenzl
2. Oyen RH, Van Poppel HP, Ameye FE, et al. Lymph node staging of localized prostatic carcinoma with cT and cT-guided fine-needle aspiration biopsy: Prospective study of 285 patients. *Radiology* 1994; 190(2): 315–322.
3. Barentsz JO, Engelbrecht MR, Witjes JA, et al. MR imaging of the male pelvis. *Eur Radiol* 1999; 9(9): 1722–1736.

Q4. Answer A

Multiple genetic and epigenetic alterations have been described in bladder cancer, including those that affect signal transduction, the cell cycle, invasion, angiogenesis and apoptosis.

Most genetic events to date have been identified in high-grade and muscle-invasive bladder cancer. Many of these events are also found in CIS, confirming the likely progression to muscle-invasive TCC via CIS.

Chromosome 9 loss of heterozygosity (LOH) is found in found in more than 50% of all bladder tumours regardless of stage and grade. Current evidence suggests that genetic alterations on chromosome 9q are an early event in bladder tumour formation. Other chromosomal alterations are loss of 17p, 3p, 13q, 18q and 10q. These are noted more frequently in high than in low grade and stage disease.

The key tumour suppressor genes altered in bladder cancer are TP53 and RB1, pathways that control the cell cycle. (P53 is a classic tumour suppressor gene and in its mutated form it is overtly stabilised and hence it is overexpressed in invasive TCC). TP53 gene is the most commonly mutated gene in high-grade muscle-invasive urothelial cancer. The TP53, retinoblastoma (RB), PTEN genes and loss of chromosome 17 are all associated with high-grade cancer. Alterations in TP53, RB and PTEN are poor prognostic indicators.

Several known oncogenes are altered in TCC. Activating point mutations of FGFR3 have been identified in approximately 40% of bladder tumours overall. Mutant FGFR3 is predicted to activate the RAS-MAP kinase pathway.

Further Reading

1. Bryan RT, Billingham LJ, Wallace DM. Molecular pathways in bladder cancer part 1&2. *BJU Int* 2005; 95(4): 485–496.

2. Knowles MA. Novel therapeutic targets in bladder cancer: Mutations and expression of FGF receptors. *Future Oncol* 2008; 4: 71–83.

Q5. Answer B

Photodynamic diagnosis (PDD) is performed using filtered blue light after intravesical instillation of a photosensitiser 5-Aminolaevulinic acid (ALA) or hexa-aminolaevulinic acid (HAL). The additional detection rate with PDD for all tumours is about 20% and about 23% for CIS.

The EAU guidelines recommend that if the equipment is available, fluorescence guided (PDD) biopsy should be performed when bladder CIS is suspected (e.g., positive urine cytology, recurrent tumour with previous history of a high-grade lesion).

Further Reading

1. Kausch I, Sommerauer M, Montorsi F, et al. Photodynamic diagnosis in non-muscle-invasive bladder cancer: A systematic review and cumulative analysis of prospective studies. *Eur Urol* 2010; 57(4): 595–606.

Q6. Answer C

The effect of early instillation can be explained by the destruction of circulating tumour cells free within the bladder immediately after TUR, or as an ablative effect (chemoresection) of the residual tumour cells at the resection site. In all single instillation studies, the instillation was administered within 24 hours. In absolute values, the reduction was 11.7% (from 48.4% to 36.7%), which implies a 24.2% decrease in the corresponding relative risk. The majority (80%) of patients in this EORTC meta-analysis showing the benefit of single, immediate instillation of intravesical chemotherapy after TURBT had a single tumour.

No prospective data are available showing that the single instillation significantly reduces recurrence rates in patients with recurrent tumours. Nevertheless, there is significant evidence from one subgroup analysis that an immediate instillation might have an impact on the repeat instillation regimen for treatment of patients who are at intermediate- and high-risk of recurrence.

Immediate instillation of chemotherapy has no reported influence on the progression rate or overall survival of patients with NMIBC. Mitomycin C, epirubicin and doxorubicin have all shown a beneficial effect, and none is superior.

Further Reading

1. Sylvester RJ, Oosterlinck W, van der Meijden AP. A single immediate postoperative instillation of chemotherapy decreases the risk of recurrence in patients with stage Ta T1 bladder cancer: A meta-analysis of published results of randomized clinical trials. *J Urol* 2004; 171(6 Pt 1): 2186–2190.

2. Kaasinen E, Rintala E, Hellstrom P, et al. FinnBladder Group. Factors explaining recurrence in patients undergoing chemoimmunotherapy regimens for frequently recurring superficial bladder carcinoma. *Eur Urol* 2002; 42(2): 167–174.

Q7. Answer C

BCG is an attenuated mycobacterium developed as a vaccine for tuberculosis that has demonstrated antitumour activity in several different cancers including urothelial cancers. BCG is stored in refrigeration and reconstituted from a lyophilised powder. Connaught, Tice, Armand Frappier, Pasteur, Tokyo and RIVM strains all arise from a common original strain developed at the Pasteur Institute. Treatments are generally begun a minimum of two weeks after tumour resection, allowing time for re-epithelialization, which minimises the potential for intravasation of live bacteria. For the same reason, a urinalysis is usually performed immediately before instillation to further ensure a diminished probability of systemic uptake of BCG. In the event of a traumatic catheterisation, the treatment should be delayed for several days to one week, depending on the extent of injury. After instillation, the patient should try and retain the solution for at least two hours however this is not always possible due to urgency and pain. Fluid, diuretic and caffeine restriction before instillation is essential to limit dilution of the agent with urine and to facilitate retention of the agent for two hours. Patients are instructed to clean their toilet with bleach after voiding and flushing. The original regimen described by Morales included a percutaneous dose, which was discontinued after success using a similar intravesical regimen.

Q8. Answer A

Apart from the B–D above, the limits of dissection of the standard pelvic lymphadenectomy includes the genitofemoral nerve laterally, not the obturator nerve. Many researchers now recommend an extended lymphadenectomy with the cephalad limits of dissection extending up to the aortic bifurcation and including caudally the presacral nodes. Not only does an extended lymph node dissection provide additional data for tumour staging, but survival might also be improved by this technique. Removal of more than 15 lymph nodes has been postulated to be both sufficient for the evaluation of the lymph node status as well as beneficial for overall survival in retrospective studies.

Further Reading

1. Ghoneim MA, Abol-Enein H. Lymphadenectomy with cystectomy: Is it necessary and what is its extent? *Eur Urol* 2004; 46(4): 457–461.

2. Wright JL, Lin DW, Porter MP. The association between extent of lymphadenectomy and survival among patients with lymph node metastases undergoing radical cystectomy. *Cancer* 2008; 112: 2332–2333.

Q9. Answer D

Patients with significantly decreased renal function are at increased risk of developing chronic acidosis and metabolic abnormalities with a continent diversion. This is due to the reabsorption of electrolytes by the bowel mucosa. There is no exact renal function cut-off below which continent urinary reconstruction should not be performed, but as a general guide, one should generally avoid it if the GFR is <50 mL/min. Abnormal GFR, hydronephrosis, previous bowel surgery with or without adjuvant chemotherapy and/or external beam radiation to the pelvis are not absolute but relative contra-indications for a neobladder. Involvement of the bladder neck is considered an absolute contraindication in both sexes. Quality of life surveys have not shown one type of urinary diversion to be superior over another. Most patients are reasonably well adapted socially, physically and psychologically to their diversion. The key to this adaptation is appropriate and realistic preoperative education. Quality of life surveys have often been underpowered or affected by selection bias. Most such studies in patients with continent urinary diversion suffer from major methodological problems. Unfortunately, there is not a single RCT within the field of urinary diversion. Almost all studies are of Level 3 evidence good-quality retrospective studies, or case series, or Level 4 evidence including expert opinion.

Q10. Answer B

Metabolic consequences of the use of bowel for urinary diversion are mainly related to bowel type and length. Considering complications of urinary contact with bowel, the length of time urine is retained, concentration of urinary solutes, urinary pH and osmolality are also important. In an ileal conduit, hydrogen is normally secreted into the lumen in exchange for sodium, whereas bicarbonate is secreted into the lumen in exchange for chloride. In the presence of diluted or hypo-osmolar urine, often seen in the early postoperative period due to low salt intake, one may see a hypovolemic salt-losing state with subsequent acidosis, hyperchloremia and hypokalaemia. Mild metabolic acidosis may be expected in up to 15% of patients after ileal conduit diversion. Due to increased urine contact time and surface the incidence of metabolic acidosis in orthotopic diversions is greater by up to 50%. The principal mechanism leading to the production of acidosis is thought to be ammonium reabsorption in hyperosmolar urine. Chloride and sodium are absorbed, pH in reservoir increases and volume decreases. Absorption of ammonium chloride leads to a hyperchloremic acidosis. Over time, chronic acidosis can lead to bone demineralisation because excess protons in the serum would be buffered against bone minerals. Acidosis may also cause osteoclast activation and potential impairment of vitamin D synthesis. It is important to recognise the clinical signs of metabolic acidosis, such as nausea, lack of appetite, fatigue, weakness and ultimately vomiting. Patients with impaired hepatic and renal function, large bowel surface and long urine-bowel contact are at increased risk of developing this disorder. One should have a high index of suspicion if patients with urinary diversions have non-specific illnesses. Acidosis and electrolyte disturbance should be excluded early. Normal serum pH and bicarbonate do not exclude a severely compensated metabolic acidosis, and blood gas analysis and body weight measurements are required. But many metabolic effects may be subtle and only recognised with continued follow-up (particularly of patients at risk). Metabolic acidosis can be best detected by regular blood gas analysis.

The terminal ileum is the sole site of vitamin B12 and of bile acid absorption. If more than 100 cm of distant ileum is resected, lipid malabsorption and therefore also fat-soluble vitamins (A, D, E and K) malabsorption will occur. All patients should be monitored regularly for B12 deficiency following the use of terminal ileum for urinary diversion. If deficiency is confirmed, lifelong supplementation with monthly intramuscular injection is required. The morbidity of radical cystectomy and urinary diversion is up to 75% diversion related.

EMQs – ANSWERS

Q11. Answer B

Q12. Answer D

Q13. Answer H

Nephrogenic adenoma is a rare tumour caused by chronic irritation of the urothelium. It arises from a variety of sources, including trauma, previous surgery, renal transplantation, intravesical chemotherapy, stones, catheters and infection. Nephrogenic adenoma is composed of glandular-appearing tubules similar to renal tubules that involve the mucosa and submucosa of the bladder. These structures are covered by cuboidal cells with clear or eosinophilic cytoplasm with cytologically normal nuclei. The lesion may be vascular, which explains the presence of gross haematuria in most cases. The most frequent presenting symptom is visible haematuria, often in conjunction with a urinary tract infection. Treatment consists of transurethral resection and elimination of the chronic irritation.

Epithelial metaplasia is the focal areas of transformed urothelium with normal nuclear and cellular architecture surrounded by normal urothelium usually located on the trigone and composed of squamous (squamous metaplasia) or glandular (glandular metaplasia) cells. Squamous metaplasia often has a knobbly appearance and is covered by white, flaky, easily disrupted material lying on the trigone. Glandular metaplasia appears as clumps of raised red areas that appear inflammatory and are often confused for cancer. There are no racial differences, and squamous metaplasia is more common in women of childbearing age. Spinal cord injury is associated with squamous metaplasia most likely from catheter trauma and urinary tract infections. Glandular metaplasia can extensively involve the bladder, particularly the trigone.

Leukoplakia of the bladder is similar to squamous metaplasia with the addition of keratin deposition that appears as a white flaky substance floating in the bladder. Leukoplakia occurs in other organs that are covered by squamous epithelium and is often premalignant. However, cytogenetic studies on bladder leukoplakia are consistent with a benign lesion, and no treatment is necessary.

An inverted papilloma is a benign proliferative lesion that is associated with chronic inflammation or bladder outlet obstruction and can be located throughout the bladder but most commonly on the trigone, comprising less than 1% of all bladder tumours. Inverted papillomas demonstrate an inverted growth pattern composed of anastomosing islands of histologically and cytologically normal urothelial cells invaginating from the surface urothelium into the lamina propria but not into the muscularis propria. When diagnosed according to strictly defined criteria (e.g., lack of cytologic atypia), inverted papillomas behave in a benign fashion with only a 1% incidence of tumour recurrence. Transurethral resection is the treatment of choice.

Leiomyomas are the most common nonepithelial benign tumour of the bladder composed of benign smooth muscle. These tumours occur most commonly in women of childbearing age and are histologically similar to leiomyomas of the uterus. Leiomyomas appear as smooth indentations of the bladder and can be confused with a bladder tumour except for the normal urothelium overlying the tumour. Imaging, especially with magnetic resonance imaging (MRI), can confirm the diagnosis and spare invasive procedures. Surgical resection is required if the leiomyoma is large or painful.

Cystitis cystica and/or glandularis is a common finding in normal bladders, usually associated with inflammation or chronic obstruction. These benign tumours represent cystic nests that are lined by columnar or cuboidal cells and are generally associated with proliferation of von Brunn's nests. Cystitis glandularis can be associated with pelvic lipomatosis and may occupy the majority of the bladder. Cystitis glandularis may develop into or coexist with intestinal metaplasia, which are benign tumours characterised by goblet cells that are histologically similar to colonic epithelium. There have been a few case reports of cystitis glandularis transforming into adenocarcinoma, and therefore, regular endoscopic evaluation of patients with these entities is recommended. The most common presenting feature of cystitis cystica or glandularis is irritative voiding symptoms and haematuria.

Urothelial papilloma is a benign proliferative growth in the bladder that is composed of delicate stalks lined by normal-appearing urothelium. Papillomas may recur, but they do not progress or invade.

Q14. Answer E

Q15. Answer B

Q16. Answer C

Sarcomas are the most common mesenchymal tumour of the bladder but comprise less than 1% of all bladder cancers. Sub classification of sarcoma is based on histologic variations, depending on the specific malignant cell type. Leiomyosarcoma is the most common histologic subtype, followed by rhabdomyosarcoma and then, rarely, angiosarcoma, osteosarcoma and carcinosarcoma. The male-to-female ratio is 2:1, and the average age at presentation is in the sixth decade of life. There are no clear agents that cause bladder sarcomas, although there is an association with pelvic radiation and systemic chemotherapy for other malignancies. Importantly, bladder sarcomas are not smoking-related. The majority of sarcomas are high-grade. The most common presenting symptom is visible haematuria. Transurethral resection of the tumour, which may appear to have normal overlying urothelium, is necessary for diagnosis along with abdominal and chest imaging. The grade of the sarcoma is the primary prognostic factor and incorporated into the overall sarcoma staging system. Treatment for localised disease includes radical cystectomy. The overall five-year disease-free survival rate for leiomyosarcoma of the bladder is 52%–62%. Active chemotherapeutic regimens are lacking for bladder sarcomas, but doxorubicin, ifosfamide and cisplatin are the most effective agents. The most common site for metastatic disease is lung, followed by bone, liver and, rarely, soft tissue organs.

Primary signet ring cell carcinoma of the bladder is extremely rare, occupying less than 1% of all epithelial bladder neoplasms. Signet ring cell carcinoma can be of urachal origin and directly extend into the bladder. These tumours generally present as high-grade, high-stage tumours and have a uniformly poor prognosis. The primary treatment is radical cystectomy.

Small-cell carcinoma primarily arises in the lung, but can occur in extra pulmonary sites, including the bladder, prostate and colon. Small-cell carcinoma of the bladder should be considered and treated as metastatic disease, even if there is no radiologic evidence of disease outside the bladder. Small-cell carcinoma of the bladder accounts for much less than 1% of all primary bladder tumours. The tumour affects men older than 70 years, and there is a slightly higher prevalence in smokers. The origin of extra pulmonary small-cell carcinoma is unclear but may be related to multipotential stem cells that can develop into small-cell carcinoma within extra pulmonary organs. The most common presenting symptom is visible haematuria; however, local irritation and pain are relatively frequent. At transurethral resection the mass is indistinguishable from urothelial carcinoma, and resection is required to make a histologic diagnosis. A variety of chemotherapeutic regimens have been used, but carboplatin or cisplatin and etoposide is the current treatment of choice. It is common to have a complete response from initial chemotherapy; however, clinical relapse occurs in greater than 80% of cases. Although chemoradiation therapy is the primary treatment for small-cell carcinoma of the bladder, experience combining chemotherapy with radical cystectomy for primary small-cell cancers of the bladder has shown equal, or perhaps better, local control and disease-free survival than found with chemo radiation. However, with 5-year cancer-specific survival rates of 16%–18% with chemo radiation or chemotherapy and radical cystectomy, respectively, the primary method to improve survival will be more effective systemic therapy.

Chronic infection with *Schistosoma haematobium* leads to squamous cell cancer of the bladder. The *Schistosoma* ova are deposited in the wall of the bladder and produce chronic inflammation that converts the urothelium to a squamous cell epithelium. Squamous cell epithelium has a much greater proliferation rate, and, with the presence of chronic inflammation, over time this greater proliferation rate leads to cancer formation. In addition, chronic infection with *Schistosoma haematobium* converts nitrates to nitrites and subsequently to nitrosamines, which are known bladder carcinogens.

Spinal cord–injured patients are also at risk for developing squamous cell carcinoma, most likely because of chronic catheter irritation and infection. Older studies have suggested a 2.5%–10% incidence of squamous cell carcinoma in the spinal cord-injured population, with a mean delay of 17 years after the spinal cord injury. More recent analysis of the association of spinal cord injury and bladder cancer formation has shown a remarkably lower risk of bladder cancer formation of 0.38%, most likely because of better catheter care. This supports the concept that chronic infection and foreign bodies can lead to bladder cancer formation.

Q17. Answer G

Q18. Answer D

Q19. Answer C

Numerous urinary molecular markers for bladder cancer diagnosis have been developed. Most commercially available urinary markers are slightly more sensitive than cytology but lack specificity. The sensitivity of tests can be improved by their combination. Current impediments to their routine usage in clinical practice include their cost effectiveness. It is generally accepted that none of the tests can replace cystoscopy to investigate haematuria presently.

Only NMP22 and BTA stat are point-of-care tests. Microsatellite analysis, gene microarray, UroVysion and Survivin are expensive and laborious.

BTA has limited role because of its high false positive rate and low sensitivity for low-grade tumour. While the BTA stat test is a point of care marker, BTA TRAK is not.

UroVysion uses fluorescence in situ hybridisation (FISH) which is a cell-based assay containing probes to the centromeres of chromosomes 3, 7 and 17 and to the 9p21 locus.

Nuclear matrix protein 22 Overall sens = 49%–68%, Overall spec = 85%–87%.

BTA stat Overall sens = 57%–83%, Overall spec = 68%–85%.

Q20. Answer B

Q21. Answer A

Q22. Answer D

The BOXIT was a phase 3 trial whose main objective was to determine if the addition of the oral COX-2 inhibitors Celecoxib to standard therapy was more effective in terms of disease recurrence at three years compared with standard therapy alone for the treatment of non-muscle-invasive TCC of the bladder in intermediate- or high-risk groups. It is inferred that Celecoxib was not shown to reduce the risk of recurrence in intermediate- or high-risk non-muscle-invasive bladder cancer, although celecoxib was associated with delayed time to recurrence in pT1 NMIBC patients.

Primary outcome measures being studied in the HYMN trial are disease-free survival and complete-response rate at 3 months. Patients will receive six weekly induction instillations of hyperthermia plus mitomycin (HM), followed by a six week pause and a cystoscopy assessment. If disease free then they will proceed to maintenance HM consisting of one instillation of HM every six weeks for the first year and one instillation every eight weeks for the second year, with further treatment in those disease-free at 24 months at the discretion of the clinician. Each instillation is divided into two 30-minute cycles each with 20 mg mitomycin dissolved in 50 mL of sterile water. Bladder hyperthermia (42°C ± 2°C) will be delivered in combination with each instillation of mitomycin. Control arm patients will receive a second course of BCG therapy. This will consist of six consecutive weekly instillations of BCG followed by maintenance therapy. Maintenance consists of three consecutive weekly instillations of BCG at 3, 6, 12, 18 and 24 months, with further treatment for those disease-free at 24 months at the discretion of the clinician.

The ODMIT-C was a prospective, randomised, non-blinded trial undertaken in 46 British centres between July 2000 and December 2006. The study recruited 284 patients with no previous or concurrent history of bladder cancer undergoing nephroureterectomy for suspected UUTUC. It looked at the value of a single dose of intravesical mitomyzin in preventing the development of bladder tumours following nephroureterectomy for transitional cell carcinoma of the upper urinary tract. The results were published in *European Urology* in October 2011 and it was shown that a single postoperative dose of intravesical reduced the risk of a bladder tumour within the first year following nephroureterectomy. The absolute reduction in risk was 11%, the relative reduction in risk was 40%, and the number needed to treat to prevent one bladder tumour was nine.

Q23. Answer C

Q24. Answer A

Q25. Answer F

UUT-UCC are uncommon and account for only 5%–10% of urothelial carcinomas (bladder tumours account for 90%–95% of urothelial carcinomas). The natural history of UUT-UCC differs from that of bladder cancer: 60% are invasive at diagnosis compared with only 15% of bladder tumours.

TNM classification (2017) for Upper Urinary Tract – Urothelial Cell Carcinoma

T Primary tumour		
	Tx	Primary tumour cannot be assessed
	T0	No evidence of primary tumour
	Ta	Non-invasive papillary carcinoma
	Tis	Carcinoma in situ
	T1	Tumour invades subepithelial connective tissue
	T2	Tumour invades muscularis
	T3	(Renal pelvis) tumour invades beyond muscularis into peripelvic fat or renal parenchyma
		(Ureter) tumour invades beyond muscularis into periureteric fat
	T4	Tumour invades adjacent organs or through the kidney into perinephric fat
N Regional lymph nodes		
	Nx	Regional lymph nodes cannot be assessed
	N0	No regional lymph node metastasis
	N1	Metastasis in a single lymph node 2 cm or less in the greatest dimension
	N2	Metastasis in a single lymph node more than 2 cm, or multiple lymph nodes
M Distant metastasis		
	M0	No distant metastasis
	M1	Distant metastasis

CHAPTER 8: RENAL CANCER

Nilay Patel (deceased), Vinodh Murali and David Cranston

MCQs

Q1. Which of the following is NOT a recognised risk factor for the development of renal carcinoma?
A. Hypertension
B. Diabetes
C. Obesity
D. Smoking
E. Haemodialysis

Q2. A 67-year-old man is noted to have an incidental small renal mass in his left kidney whilst undergoing investigation for rectal bleeding. An upper pole tumour is noted to be entirely endophytic and 38 mm in maximal dimension. The tumour lies anteriorly within the upper pole and is in contact with the collecting system though does not cross the inter-polar lines. What would be the R.E.N.A.L. nephrometry score of this tumour?
A. 7a
B. 8a
C. 9p
D. 10a
E. 12p

Q3. Von Hippel–Lindau disease is associated with mutations on which gene locus?
A. 1q42
B. 3p25
C. 7q31
D. 9q34
E. 17p11

Q4. Which one of the following statements regarding active surveillance of T1a small renal masses is CORRECT?
A. Active surveillance is the recommended treatment of choice for low grade
B. Clear cell renal cell carcinoma

C. Malignant tumours can grow at a faster rate than benign lesions.
D. The risk of metastatic progression on active surveillance is the same as for all other treatment options.
E. Masses have an average annual growth rate of 0.75 cm/year.
F. Less than 10% of SRMs demonstrate negative or zero growth rates.

Q5. Which one of the following statements regarding locally advanced renal cell cancer is CORRECT?
A. T3b (TNM classification 2017) RCC have tumour thrombus in the IVC above the diaphragm.
B. The 5-year cancer-specific survival rates for T3b renal cell cancers treated by surgery (TNM classification 2017) is 40%.
C. The ipsilateral adrenal gland should be excised with the kidney when there is an upper pole renal tumour.
D. 5-year cancer-specific survival rates are the same for tumour thrombus within the IVC below the diaphragm compared with invasion of the IVC wall by tumour thrombus.
E. Extended regional lymph node dissection at the time of nephrectomy significantly increases cancer-specific survival.

Q6. Which one of the following statements regarding ablative therapies for renal cell cancer is CORRECT?
A. Cryotherapy is the gold standard treatment for a T1a renal cell cancer in a fit patient.
B. The commonest complication following cryotherapy of small renal masses (<4 cm) is pain or paraesthesia at the probe insertion site

C. High-intensity frequency ultrasound (HIFU) is a recognised treatment for small renal tumours.

D. Local recurrence rates are higher for cryotherapy compared to RFA for T1a renal cell cancers.

E. The radiographic measures of post ablative success following cryoablation and radiofrequency ablation are well-established.

Q7. Which one of the following statements regarding renal biopsy is CORRECT?

A. Percutaneous needle biopsy of renal masses is diagnostic in approximately 95% of cases in contemporary series.

B. Repeat percutaneous renal mass biopsy is diagnostic in 50% of cases in contemporary series.

C. Complications occur in 15% of percutaneous renal mass biopsies.

D. Success rates of percutaneous renal mass biopsies are not operator dependent.

E. Contemporary series show a 0.1% tumour seeding rate in the biopsy tract following percutaneous renal mass biopsy.

Q8. Which one of the following statements regarding laparoscopic nephrectomy is CORRECT?

A. Laparoscopic nephrectomy is the gold standard treatment for T1b renal cell carcinomas.

B. Retroperitoneal approach for a laparoscopic nephrectomy offers significant advantages over the transperitoneal approach.

C. Port site metastasis have not been reported following laparoscopic radical nephrectomy for RCC.

D. Long-term (10 years) oncological outcomes for laparoscopic radical nephrectomy vs open radical nephrectomy for T1 & T2 RCC are equivalent.

E. Trocar injuries are the commonest complication associated with laparoscopic nephrectomy.

Q9. Which one of the following statements regarding the surgical management of metastatic renal cancer is CORRECT?

A. Cytoreductive nephrectomy prolongs progression free survival in combination with tyrosine kinase inhibitors (TKI's) in metastatic RCC.

B. 2% of patients with metastatic RCC will be cured when treated with cytoreductive nephrectomy and TKIs.

C. Metastasectomy can cure up to 20% of patients with a solitary RCC metastases.

D. Presence of sarcomatoid features in a solitary renal cell recurrence is a good prognostic factor.

E. Abnormal serum lactate dehydrogenase and alkaline phosphatase at the time of a local renal cell recurrence are worse prognostic factors.

Q10. Which of the following molecular biomarkers improves the accuracy of the SSIGN scoring system in predicting cancer specific survival in renal cell carcinoma?

A. HIF
B. CA9
C. p53
D. IMP3
E. VEGF

Q11. The ONLY primary renal tumour which expresses HMB-45 is:

A. AML
B. Clear cell RCC
C. Oncocytoma
D. Renal medullary carcinoma
E. Chromophobe RCC

Q12. The MOST common form of RCC in patients in end-stage renal disease and in patients on dialysis is:

A. Clear cell RCC
B. Papillary RCC
C. Chromophobe RCC
D. Collecting duct RCC
E. Tubulocystic RCC

Q13. All of the following features are TRUE about metastatic RCC, except:
A. Metastases occur by lymphatic and hematogenous spread with equal frequency.
B. Regional lymph nodes are the most common site of metastasis.
C. Metastasis usually involves multiple sites rather than single site.
D. Risk of metastasis on presentation for pT1b tumours is 16%.
E. If metastasis develops after nephrectomy for an M0 renal cancer, they usually occur within one year of surgery.

Q14. Which of the following is TRUE about tuberous sclerosis?
A. The classic triad of tuberous sclerosis include adenoma sebaceum, seizures and AML.
B. 10% of patients with TS develop RCC.
C. TS is an autosomal dominant disease caused by mutation of TSC1 gene (chromosome 16) and TSC2 gene (chromosome 9).
D. Adenoma sebaceum usually develop after puberty.
E. The classic triad is seen in only 30% of the patients.

Q15. The following risk factors are included in BOTH MSKCC risk models and IMDC risk models, except:
A. Karnofsky performance <80
B. Anaemia
C. Neutrophilia
D. Hypercalcemia
E. Time from diagnosis to treatment <12 months

Q16. The first line treatment option for IMDC poor risk metastatic RCC is:
A. Pazopanib
B. Ipilimumab/nivolumab
C. Sorafenib
D. Temsirolimus
E. Axitinib

Q17. All of the following are FALSE about Bosniak cysts, except:
A. Hyperdense cysts always need follow-up.
B. Nodular calcification without enhancement indicates Type 3 cyst.
C. Type 1 cysts are malignant in 10% of cases.
D. All type 2 cysts need follow-up for up to 5 years.
E. Biopsy should always be considered in any renal cyst before contemplating on nephrectomy.

Q18. The MOST common site of distant recurrence after curative treatment for primary RCC is:
A. Spine
B. Lung
C. Liver
D. Brain
E. Adrenal

Q19. All of the following are factors that INCREASE the risk of hyperfiltration injury, except:
A. High protein diet
B. Poorly controlled DM
C. HTN
D. Use of statins
E. Removal of more than 75% of functional renal mass

Q20. All of the following are prognostic nomograms for localised RCC, except:
A. MSKCC nomogram
B. UISS model
C. SSIGN prognostic model
D. A and B
E. A and C

EMQs

Q21–25. Hereditary RCC
  A. Von Hippel–Lindau disease
  B. Hereditary papillary RCC
  C. Hereditary leiomyomatosis RCC
  D. Birt–Hogg–Dubé syndrome
  E. Lynch syndrome

Choose the most appropriate response from the list above. Each option may be used once, more than once or not at all.

Q21. Associated with pheochromocytoma

Q22. Associated with chromophobe rcc

Q23. Characterised by micro-satellite instability

Q24. Mutations in the c-met oncogene

Q25. Associated with lung cysts and pneumothoraces

Q26–30. Targeted therapies mode of action/side effects
  A. Sunitinib
  B. Sorafenib
  C. Bevacizumab
  D. Temsirolimus
  E. Interleukin-2
  F. Pazopanib

Choose the most appropriate response from the list above. Each option may be used once, more than once or not at all.

Q26. Monoclonal anti-body to VEGF

Q27. First line treatment for patients with risk stratified as MSKCC – high-risk

Q28. Hypertension is observed in 30% of patients following therapy

Q29. Inhibitor of mammalian target of rapamycin (mTOR)

Q30. Inhibitor of the VEGFR1

Q31–35. TNM classification for renal cancer
  A. T1aN0M0
  B. T2aN0M0
  C. T2bN1M0
  D. T2bN2M0
  E. T3aN0M0
  F. T3bN0M0
  G. T4N0M0

Choose the most appropriate response from the list above. Each option may be used once, more than once or not at all.

Q31. 5.5 cm RCC with extension into the ipsi-lateral adrenal gland. No nodes or distant metastases.

Q32. 11 cm RCC with a 3.5 cm para-aortic lymph node with no distant metastases.

Q33. 2 cm RCC with invasion into the renal sinus veins. No nodes or distant metastases.

Q34. 8 cm RCC with invasion into the inferior vena cava up to the level of the hepatic veins. No nodes or distant metastases.

Q35. 10.2 cm RCC with invasion into the peri-renal fat. No nodes or distant metastases.

Q36–40. Pathology of renal cancer
  A. Papillary Cell (Type 1)
  B. Papillary cell (Type 2)
  C. Clear cell
  D. Chromophobe
  E. Collecting duct
  F. Medullary carcinoma

Choose the most appropriate response from the list above. Each option may be used once, more than once or not at all.

Q36. Tumours are composed of small cells with scanty cytoplasm, arranged in a single layer on the papillary basement membrane that stains positive for CK7 was strong or moderate in more than 75% of cases

Q37. Strongly associated with sickle cell disease

Q38. Cells are lipid and glycogen rich and stain positive for CD10 in more than 90% of cases

Q39. Stains strongly for Hale's colloidal iron

Q40. Tumours can appear as cystic masses

Q41–45. A 63-year-old man is diagnosed with a 35 mm solid enhancing lesion in his right kidney. He opts to under an open partial nephrectomy.
- A. 65
- B. 30
- C. 20
- D. 35
- E. 6
- F. 11

Choose the most appropriate response from the list above. Each option may be used once, more than once or not at all.

Q41. The percentage of patients who develop an eGFR of less than 60 mL/min per 1.73 m^2 (CKD 3–5) after a partial nephrectomy.

Q42. What is the optimal upper limit of warm ischaemia time following hilar clamping for a partial nephrectomy?

Q43. What is the optimal upper limit of cold ischaemia time following hilar clamping for a partial nephrectomy?

Q44. The percentage of patients who develop major urological following an open partial nephrectomy.

Q45. What percentage of patients develops disease recurrence following a positive surgical margin after a partial nephrectomy?

MCQs – ANSWERS

Q1. Answer B

Hypertension and the use of anti-hypertensive medications are associated with an increased risk of RCC. Studies have shown a clear dose-response relationship between elevated blood pressure and an increased risk of RCC. The independent contributions of hypertension and the use of antihypertensive medications have been difficult to separate, as most studies are based on a diagnosis of hypertension which is inevitably associated with treatment with antihypertensive drugs. Better control of blood pressure may lower RCC risk.

Whilst diabetes mellitus (DM) type 2 has been shown to be associated with an increased risk of several cancers, no significant increased risk has been demonstrated between DM and RCC [1].

Obesity has been established as a risk factor for RCC in a number of studies. A meta-analysis [2], demonstrated that the risk of RCC increased with elevated body mass index (BMI), with summary risk estimates (per 5 kg/m^2 increase in BMI) of 1.24 in men and 1.34 in women. It has been proposed that the increased risk of RCC in obese patients may be due to increased exposure to oestrogens and androgens.

Cigarette smoking is a well-established risk factor for RCC. A meta-analysis of 24 studies showed that a history of smoking increases the risk of RCC compared to never smoking. Though the association between smoking and RCC is relatively weak, a dose-response relationship has been shown.

Acquired renal cystic disease (ARCD) arises predominantly in patients with end-stage renal disease treated with haemodialysis. The incidence of RCC in ARCD is up to six times higher than in the general population. The risk of developing RCC does not appear to decrease after renal transplantation.

Q2. Answer B

The R.E.N.A.L nephrometry scoring system was introduced by Kutikov et al. [3] as a standardised scoring system to characterise renal tumour anatomy and complexity in a reproducible, quantifiable manner. The aim of the scoring system was to allow meaningful comparisons of renal masses in clinical practice and in the urological literature. Tumours are evaluated using a 3-point scale on the basis of the following:

	1 pt	2 pts	3 pts
Radius (maximal diameter in cm)	≤4	>4 but <7	≥7
Exophytic/endophytic properties	≥50%	<50%	Entirely endophytic
Nearness of the tumour to the collecting system or sinus (mm)	≥7	>4 but <7	≤4
Anterior/posterior	No points given. Mass assigned a descriptor of a, p, or x		
Location relative to the polar lines[a]	Entirely above the upper or below the polar line	Lesion crosses polar line	>50% of mass is across polar line (a) or mass crosses the axial renal midline (b) or mass is entirely between the polar lines (c)

[a] suffix 'h' assigned if the tumour touches the main renal artery or vein.

The above tumours would be scored as; R = 1, E = 3, N = 3, a, L = 1, giving a nephrometry score of 8a.

R.E.N.A.L nephrometry scores have been used to develop a nomogram that helps to predict the likelihood of malignant and high-grade pathology of an enhancing renal mass. Increasing tumour complexity as determined by nephrometry score is associated with an increased likelihood of major complications. Two alternative scoring systems have also been developed (PADUA and C-index) with the intention of providing a standardised descriptive system for renal masses based on radiologic findings [4].

Q3. Answer B

Von Hippel–Lindau (VHL) disease is the most common hereditary renal cancer syndrome with an incidence of 1 in 35,000 live births. VHL disease arises as a result of mutations in the Von Hippel–Lindau tumour suppressor (VHL) gene located at 3p25. Germ line mutations are present in nearly 100% of affected individuals with subsequent inactivation of the wild-type copy of the VHL gene leading to the clinical manifestation of VHL disease; clear cell renal cell carcinoma, CNS or retinal haemangioblastoma, pheochromocytoma and pancreatic cysts. RCCs are seen in up to 50% of VHL patients are often multiple and bilateral. Metastatic RCC is the most common cause of mortality in VHL patients [5].

The VHL protein acts as an E3 ubiquitin ligase and targets the alpha sub-unit of hypoxia inducible factor (HIF) for ubiquitin-mediated degradation. The inactivating mutations of both alleles of the VHL gene seen in VHL disease results in the constitutive over expression of HIF and its downstream targets VEGF, PDGF, TGF-a, erythropoietin, GLUT-1 and CA9, which in turn are key drivers of the oncogenic.

The fumarate hydratase gene is located at locus 1q42 and is associated with hereditary leiomyomatosis and RCC. 7q31 represents the locus for the c-met oncogene linked to hereditary papillary RCC. Tuberose sclerosis has been shown to arise as a result of mutations in the hamartin gene located at 9q34, whilst 17p11 is the locus for the folliculin gene which results in Birt–Hogg–Dubé syndrome.

Q4. Answer C

Active surveillance has traditionally been reserved for the treatment of T1 small renal masses in elderly patients with multiple co-morbidities or those who decline surgery. The current guidelines for the treatment of T1 renal cancer from the American Urological Association (AUA) and the European Association of Urology (EAU) both propose partial nephrectomy as the gold standard treatment option in the surgically fit patient.

A number of studies have shown that on average benign oncocytomas grow at the same rate as RCC.

Metastatic progression rates for T1a SRMs managed with AS are reported to be between 1% and 2%. Kunkle et al performed a meta-analysis of oncologic outcomes for over 6,000 SRMs and concluded that no statistically significant differences were detected in the incidence of metastatic progression regardless of whether lesions were excised, ablated or observed [6].

A meta-analysis of active surveillance for SRMs revealed a mean growth rate of 0.28 cm/year at a mean follow up of 34 months. Data from a pooled analysis by Smaldone et al demonstrated that T1a tumours have a growth rate of 0.31 cm/year [7]. Jewett et al. noted an annual growth rate of 0.13 cm/year for T1a masses in the prospective Canadian Small Renal Mass Trial.

Numerous studies have previously demonstrated a degree of variability in growth rates of T1 renal masses. Studies have demonstrated that 23%–36% of T1 SRMs have zero or negative growth rates. The pooled analysis of 880 patients with SRMs by Smaldone et al observed that metastatic progression was not observed in any patient who had negative or zero growth on follow-up, which is of great importance when counselling patients being managed with AS.

Q5. Answer B

The TNM 2017 staging classifies T3b as tumour grossly extending into the inferior vena cava *below* the diaphragm [8]. The 5-year cancer-specific survival rates for T3b renal cell cancer is 40%. The ipsilateral adrenal gland should be removed when there is evidence on CT imaging of direct invasion of the adrenal gland by the renal cell cancer or a metastasis is present in the adrenal gland that appears solitary. Tumour thrombus invading the IVC wall portends a worse prognosis (T3c staging in 2017 classification) than tumour thrombus in the IVC lumen below the diaphragm (T3b staging in 2010 classification). Radical Excision of regional para-aortic lymph nodes has not been shown to significantly improve cancer specific survival [9].

Q6. Answer B

EAU and AUA guidelines advise a partial nephrectomy in healthy patients for T1a renal cell cancers [10]. Cryotherapy and radiofrequency ablation should be reserved for carefully selected high-risk surgical patients with small renal masses <4 cm. Pain or paraesthesia at the probe insertion site is the commonest complication after cryotherapy, occurring in 7.2%. High-intensity frequency ultrasound should presently be considered an experimental treatment for small renal masses. Local recurrence rates for radiofrequency ablation are similar or higher than cryotherapy and both are significantly higher than for open partial nephrectomy [11]. The radiographic measurements of post ablative success for cryotherapy and radiofrequency ablation are not well-established presently.

Q7. Answer A

Traditionally, percutaneous renal biopsy has been criticised for the problems with non-diagnostic samples, complications and a small but real risk of tumour seeding into the biopsy tract (0.01%). Contemporary series however show a 94.5% diagnostic accuracy for percutaneous renal mass biopsies [12]. Complications rates are low at 3.5%. The Canadian small renal mass surveillance study demonstrated an 80% diagnostic accuracy when re-biopsying for a non-diagnostic initial biopsy [13]. Percutaneous renal biopsies have a learning curve and are operator dependent. No tumour seeding has been reported in the biopsy tract in contemporary series.

Q8. Answer D

The EAU and AUA guidelines recommend a partial nephrectomy should be attempted in T1b renal cell cancers where feasible though open and laparoscopic radical nephrectomies are options when partial nephrectomy is not possible. No clear benefits have been shown of performing a laparoscopic nephrectomy retroperitoneally or transperitoneally [14]. Port site metastases have been reported in a very small number of cases after laparoscopic radical nephrectomy for renal cell cancer. Both intermediate- and long-term outcomes for laparoscopic radical nephrectomy for RCC in T1 and T2 disease have been shown to be equivalent [11]. Vascular injuries and bleeding are the commonest complication seen from laparoscopic nephrectomy.

Q9. Answer E

The role of cytoreductive nephrectomy in combination with TKIs for metastatic renal cancer has been the subject of several ongoing clinical trials. There is no evidence to date of increases in progression free survival due to cytoreductive nephrectomy in combination with TKIs [15].

Sunitinib alone was not inferior to nephrectomy followed by sunitinib in patients with metastatic renal-cell carcinoma who were classified as having intermediate-risk or poor-risk disease (CARMENA). Progression-free Rate has been found to be unaffected by the sequence of cytoreductive nephrectomy and Sunitinib in patients with synchronous mRCC (EORTC – NCT01099423). There have been no reported cases of cure to date when TKIs have been combined with cytoreductive nephrectomy in metastatic renal cell cancer. Up to 50% 5-year survival rates have been reported following excision of a solitary renal cell carcinoma metastasis [16]. Positive surgical margins after resection of a local recurrence, size >5 cm of a local recurrence, presence of sarcomatoid dedifferentiation in a local recurrence and abnormal serum alkaline phosphatase/lactate dehydrogenase at the time of the local recurrence are all associated with worse prognosis.

Q10. Answer D

A number of prognostic models for patients with RCC have been developed to predict cancer specific survival. One model is the stage, size, grade and necrosis (SSIGN) score developed by the Mayo Clinic, which predicts cancer specific survival (CSS) in patients with clear cell RCC [17]. This validated scoring system scores renal tumours on the basis of the following parameters:

Parameter	Score points
Pathological tumour category	
pT1	0
pT2	1
pT3a	2
pT3b	3
pT3c	4
pT4	5
Nodal status	
Nx	0
pN0	0
pN1	2
pN2	2
Metastasis category	
M0	0
M1	4
Tumour size	
<5 cm	0
>5 cm	2

(Continued)

Parameter	Score points
Tumour grade	
1	0
2	0
3	1
4	3
Tumour necrosis	
Absent	0
Present	2

Patients can then be stratified into low-risk = 0–2 (5-year CSS = 96%–99%), intermediate-risk = 3–5 (5-year CSS = 65%–88%) and high-risk >6 (5-year CSS = 7%–55%). The use of scoring systems such as SSIGN or the UCLA devised integrated staging system (UISS), which relies on the TNM stage, Fuhrman grade and Eastern Cooperative Oncology Group Performance Status (ECOG-PS), can be used to tailor follow-up regimens and potentially identify patients that may benefit from adjuvant therapy.

A greater understanding of the molecular basis of renal carcinoma has led to the identification of a number of biomarkers that may help improve individual prognostication and risk-stratified clinical decision making.

Loss of functional VHL leads to increased expression levels of HIF in clear cell RCC.

Elevated HIF-1a levels in tumour tissue are associated with worse survival in clear cell RCC. High levels of HIF-1a or HIF-2a confer a favourable response to Sunitinib therapy in metastatic RCC.

Vascular endothelial growth factor (VEGF) plays a key role in tumour angiogenesis in RCC. In clear cell RCC VEGF expression correlates with tumour size, Fuhrman grade, tumour necrosis, tumour stage, microvessel invasion, RCC progression rate and RCC-specific survival.

Carbonic anhydrase IX (CAIX) is a HIF-1a-regulated transmembrane protein thought to assist in regulating intracellular and extracellular pH. In clear cell RCC, CAIX can establish the diagnosis as it is expressed in >80% of RCC samples and 90% of clear cell RCC specimens. High CAIX expression is associated with a better prognosis in localised RCC and mRCC.

The p53 protein plays an important role in regulating cell growth and proliferation by stopping cell cycle and inducting apoptosis in the presence of DNA damage. The prognostic role of p53 in RCC remains controversial though one study has shown that p53 over-expression was an independent predictor of metastasis-free survival in patients with localised clear cell RCC (p = 0.01).

Insulin-like growth factor II mRNA-binding protein 3 (IMP3) regulates transcription of insulin-like growth factor II. IMP3 expression was significantly associated with advanced T stage and grade, increased regional lymph node involvement, and distant metastases, tumour necrosis and sarcomatoid differentiation. In addition, multivariable, Positive IMP3 expression was independently associated with an increased risk of death from RCC even after adjusting for prognostic features comprising the SSIGN score [18].

Q11. **Answer D**

AML is the only primary renal tumour that expresses HMB 45 [19]. If a primary tumour stains positive for HMB 45, it is an AML.

Q12. Answer B

Acquired cystic kidney disease [ACKD] and a higher incidence of RCC are typical features of ESKD (end-stage kidney disease). RCCs of native end-stage kidneys are found in about 4% of patients. The lifetime risk of developing RCCs is at least 10 times higher than in the general population. Compared with sporadic RCCs, ACKDs generally are multicentric and bilateral, found in younger patients (mostly male) and are less aggressive [20, 21]. The relatively indolent outcome of tumours in ESKD is due to the mode of diagnosis and a specific ACKD related molecular pathway still to be determined. Although the histological spectrum of ACKD tumours is similar to that in sporadic RCC, the predominant form is papillary RCC [21].

Q13. Answer B

In clinical practice, 20% of patients present with metastatic disease. When a metastatic disease is discovered, a solitary metastasis is present only in 1% of cases. Metastases occur by lymphatic and hematogenous spread with equal frequency. Distant metastasis is present in >50% of patients with regional lymph node metastasis. The most common site of metastasis (most to least) is lung, bone, regional lymph nodes, liver, adrenal gland, contralateral kidney and brain. The most common site of bone metastasis is spine. Risk of metastasis on presentation for 3–4 cm, 4–7 cm, 7–10 cm and 10–15 cm renal tumours is 7%, 16%, 30% and 41%, respectively [22]. If metastasis develops after nephrectomy for an M0 renal cancer, they usually occur within one year of surgery.

Q14. Answer E

Tuberous sclerosis (TS) is an autosomal dominant disease caused by the mutation of TSC1 gene (chromosome 9) and TSC2 gene (chromosome 16). The classic triad of tuberous sclerosis (adenoma sebaceum, seizures and mental retardation) is seen in only 30% of the patients. Adenoma sebaceum are pink- or red-coloured papules usually present on nasolabial folds. They usually develop between age 4 and puberty. Urologic manifestations – renal cysts (usually develop in childhood), AML (usually B/L and multifocal) [23, 24], RCC (in 2% of patients).

Q15. Answer C

MSKCC and IMDC – The MSKCC (Motzer) criteria was developed during the cytokine era and the International Metastatic Renal Cancer Database Consortium (IMDC) risk model was established and validated to yield an accurate prognosis for patients treated in the era of targeted therapy. In IMDC risk model, neutrophilia and thrombocytosis have been added to the list of MSKCC risk factors, while LDH has been removed.

Risk factor	MSKCC risk factors	IMDC risk factors
Time from diagnosis to systemic treatment <1 year	X	X
Haemoglobin less than lower limit of normal	X	X
Calcium greater than upper limit of normal	X	X
Karnofsky <80%	X	X
LDH greater than 1.5 upper limit of normal		

(Continued)

Risk factor	MSKCC risk factors	IMDC risk factors
Neutrophil count greater than upper limit of normal		X
Platelet count greater than upper limit of normal		X

0 risk factors – favourable prognosis

1–2 risk factors – intermediate risk

>2 risk factors – poor risk

Q16. Answer B

The various lines of therapy have been outlined below (EAU guidelines 2019).

	First-line therapy	Second-line therapy	Third-line therapy
IMDC favourable-risk disease	Sunitinib or pazopanib[a]	Cabozantinib or nivolumab[a]	Cabozantinib or nivolumab[a]
IMDC intermediate- and poor-risk disease	Ipilimumab/ nivolumab[a]	Cabozantinib or VEGF-targeted therapy[a]	Cabozantinib or an alternative targeted therapy[a]
IMDC intermediate- and poor-risk disease	Cabozantinib, sunitib or pazopanib	VEGF-targeted therapy or nivolumab[a]	An alternative targeted therapy or nivolumab[a]

[a] represent strong indications

Q17. Answer B

This classification system classifies renal cysts into five categories, based on CT imaging appearance and to predict malignancy risk [25, 26].

- **Bosniak Type 1 (Benign)** – Simple benign cyst with a hairline-thin wall without septa, calcification, or solid components. Same density as water and does not enhance with contrast medium.
- **Bosniak Type II (Benign)** – Cyst that may contain a few hairline-thin septa. Fine calcification may be present in the wall or septa. Uniformly, high-attenuation lesions <3 cm in size, with sharp margins without enhancement.
- **Bosniak Type IIF (Follow-up. Some are malignant)** – These may contain more hairline-thin septa. Minimal enhancement of a hairline-thin septum or wall. Minimal thickening of the septa or wall. The cyst may contain calcification, which may be nodular and thick, with no contrast enhancement. No enhancing soft-tissue elements. Totally intrarenal, non-enhancing, high attenuation renal lesions >3 cm. Generally well-marginated.
- **Bosniak Type III (Surgery or active surveillance. More than 50% are malignant)** These are indeterminate cystic masses with thickened irregular walls or septa with enhancement.
- **Bosniak Type IV (Surgery, most are malignant)** – Clearly malignant containing enhancing soft-tissue components.

Q18. Answer B

After partial or radical nephrectomy, local recurrence in the renal fossa is rare (<2%) [27]. Recurrence in the contralateral kidney is rare (1.2%) [28]. Lung is the most common site of distant recurrence. Most recurrences occur within the first three years of treatment [29].

Q19. Answer D

When functional renal tissue is removed, glomerular hyperfiltration occurs in the remaining tissue to restore filtration capacity. Prolonged glomerular hyperfiltration may lead to renal injury in the form of focal segmental glomerulosclerosis and progressive renal failure [30].

This may take more than 10 years to develop. Proteinuria is the harbinger of hyperfiltration renal injury [31]. Risk factors for development of hyperfiltration injury include high protein diet, poorly controlled DM, HTN, use of steroids, obesity, hyperlipidaemia and removal of more than 75% of functional renal mass.

Q20. Answer A

The prognostic models in RCC vary according to the stage and are described below (EAU guidelines 2019).

1. **Localised RCC**

   a. USS model – TNM stage, ECOG performance status, Fuhrman grade

   b. SSIGN model – TNM stage, Fuhrman grade, tumour necrosis, tumour size

   c. Karakiewicz's nomogram – TNM stage, RCC related symptoms, Fuhrman grade, tumour size

2. **Metastatic RCC**

   a. MSKCC model – Karnofsky performance status, delay between diagnosis and treatment, Hb, corrected calcium, LDH, delay between diagnosis and treatment

   b. Heng model – Karnofsky performance status, delay between diagnosis and treatment, Hb, corrected calcium, neutrophil, platelets

EMQs – ANSWERS

Q21. Answer A

Q22. Answer D

Q23. Answer E

Q24. Answer B

Q25. Answer D

Numerous hereditary kidney cancer syndromes have been described which all demonstrate an autosomal dominant inheritance pathway. The application of molecular biological techniques has identified a number of defective genes that ordinarily appear to share common cellular metabolic pathways [32].

Von Hippel–Lindau (VHL) disease arises as a result of silencing mutations in the VHL gene (3p25). The VHL protein regulates intra-cellular levels of hypoxia inducible factor (HIF). Dysfunctional VHL as occurs in VHL disease results in the constitutive over expression of HIF and its downstream targets. VHL disease is associated with development of clear cell renal cell carcinoma, pheochromocytoma, retinal/CNS hemangioblastomas and pancreatic cysts.

Hereditary papillary renal cell carcinoma (HPRCC) has been linked to mutations in the MET gene (7q31), the cell surface receptor for hepatocyte growth factor. Activating mutations of MET leads to increased intracellular signalling which promotes proliferation, transformation and invasion. HPRCC is associated with the development of multi-focal, bilateral type 1 papillary renal cell carcinoma. No extra renal manifestation has been described.

Hereditary Leiomyomatosis RCC (HLRCC) arises as a result of mutations in the fumarate hydratase gene (1q42) a component of the Krebs cycle. Inactivating mutations in fumarate hydratase result in the accumulation of fumarate which in turn results in decreased degradation of HIF. HLRCC is characterised by the development of aggressive type 2 papillary RCCs, uterine leiomyoma/leiomyosarcoma and cutaneous leiomyoma/leiomyosarcomas.

Birt–Hogg–Dubé (BHD) is associated with mutations in the folliculin gene (17p11). Folliculin is a tumour suppressor gene that plays a role in signalling through the AMPK-mTOR pathways. Features of BHD include the development of multiple and bilateral RCC (chromophobe, oncocytoma, hybrid oncocytic RCC, clear cell RCC), cutaneous fibro-folliculoma, lung cysts/spontaneous pneumothoraces, colonic polyps and cancer.

Lynch syndrome or hereditary non-polyposis colorectal cancer (HNPCC) as it is now known is an autosomal dominant condition which predisposes to the development of numerous malignancies including colon, endometrium, ovary and upper urinary tract urothelial cell carcinoma. The molecular signature of HNPCC is the presence of microsatellite instability secondary to inactivating mutations of the DNA mismatch repair system [33].

Q26. Answer C

Q27. Answer D

Q28. Answer A

Q29. Answer D

Q30. Answer F

Sunitinib is a tyrosine kinase inhibitor (TKI) specific to the VEGFR2, PDGFR, FLT-3, c-KIT receptors indicated for the treatment of metastatic RCC [21]. Sunitinib therapy offers a 6-month improvement in progression free survival (11 vs 5 months) and a 5-month improvement in overall survival (26.4 vs 21.8 months) when compared with interferon therapy. The normal dosing strategy is 50 mg orally once per day for four weeks. The drug is well-tolerated with response rates of up to 40%. The most significant side effects cardiac toxicity, hypertension and hypothyroidism. Sunitinib has NICE approval for the treatment of metastatic RCC.

Sorafenib is a TKI with efficacy against VEGFR2, VEGFR3, PDGFR, FLT-3, c-KIT, CRAF and BRAF. Sorafenib treatment results in a 3-month improvement in progression free survival (5.5 vs 2.8 months) and overall survival (17.8 vs 14.3 months) compared to placebo in patients with cytokine resistant metastatic RCC. Sorafenib is administered orally at a dose of 400 mg twice per day.

Bevacizumab is a monoclonal antibody to vascular endothelial growth factor (VEGF). Combination therapy with bevacizumab and interferon prolonged progression-free survival by 5 months compared to interferon therapy alone (10.2 vs 5.4 months). Combination therapy with bevacizumab and interferon is approved as a first-line therapeutic option for metastatic RCC.

Temsirolimus is an inhibitor of mammalian inhibitor of rapamycin (mTOR) a pathway, which acts upstream of HIF. Patients with high-risk metastatic RCC as defined by the MSKCC criteria showed a 3-month overall survival benefit with temsirolimus treatment compared to interferon therapy (10.9 vs 7.3 months). The MSKCC risk stratification criteria are based upon: LDH > 1.5 normal, Haemoglobin < normal, Calcium > 2.5 mmol/L, Karnofsky Performance score and the number of metastatic site. Low risk = 0 risk factors, Intermediate risk = 1 or 2 risk factors, High risk = 3 or more of the above criteria.

Pazopanib is the latest TKI with activity against VEGFR1, VEGFR2, VEGFR3, PDGFRA, PDGFRB and c-Kit. Pazopanib therapy is well-tolerated and results in a 5-month improvement in progression-free survival for metastatic RCC (9.2 vs 4.2 months) compared to placebo. For treatment naïve patients the benefit is even greater (11.1 vs 2.8 months). Pazopanib is approved by NICE as a first line therapy for the treatment of metastatic RCC [34].

Q31. Answer G

Q32. Answer C

Q33. Answer E

Q34. Answer F

Q35. Answer E

The TNM classification developed by the International Union Against Cancer (UICC) and the American Joint Committee on Cancer (AJCC) is the standard method of staging urological malignancies. The aim of the TNM staging system is to allow effective communication of tumour characteristics, permit the evaluation of different treatment strategies, determine the selection criteria for clinical trials and ultimately aid the selection process for treating an individual patient.

The classification system for kidney cancers was revised in 2017 with modifications made to the staging of organ confined and locally invasive kidney tumours. In comparison with the 2002 staging system; (i) T2 cancers were subclassified into two subgroups based on a tumour size cut-off point of 10 cm (T2a < 10 vs. T2b > 10 cm); (ii) tumours with renal vein involvement or perinephric fat involvement were classified as T3a; (ii) tumours with adrenal involvement were classified as T4 cancers.

T –	**Primary tumour**
Tx	Primary tumour cannot be assessed
T0	No evidence of primary tumour
T1	Tumour ≤ 7 cm in greatest dimension, limited to the kidney
	• T1a Tumour ≤ 4 cm in greatest dimension, limited to the kidney
	• T1b Tumour > 4 cm but ≤ 7 cm in greatest dimension
T2	Tumour > 7 cm in greatest dimension, limited to the kidney
	• T2a Tumour > 7 cm but ≤ 10 cm in greatest dimension
	• T2b Tumours > 10 cm limited to the kidney
T3	Tumour extends into major veins or directly invades adrenal gland or perinephric tissues but not into the ipsilateral adrenal gland and not beyond Gerota's fascia
	• T3a Tumour grossly extends into the renal vein or its segmental branches or tumour invades the pelvi-calyceal system, or tumour invades perirenal and/or renal sinus (peripelvic) fat but not beyond Gerota's fascia
	• T3b Tumour grossly extends into the vena cava below the diaphragm
	• T3c Tumour grossly extends into vena cava above the diaphragm or invades the wall of the vena cava
T4	Tumour invades beyond Gerota's fascia (including contiguous extension into the ipsilateral adrenal gland)

N –	**Regional lymph nodes**
Nx	Regional lymph nodes cannot be assessed
N0	No regional lymph node metastasis
N1	Metastasis in regional lymph node
M –	**Distant metastasis**
M0	No distant metastasis
M1	Distant metastasis

TNM stage grouping
Stage I T1N0M0
Stage II T2N0M0
Stage III T3N0M0 or T1/2/3N1M0
Stage IV T4N0/1/2M0 or Any TN2M0 or any T any N M1

External validation of the revised 2009 classification was performed by Novara et al. [35]. This study showed the following 5-year CSS rates; T1a = 94.9%. T1b = 92.6%, T2a = 85.4%, T2b = 70%, T3a = 64.7%, T3b = 54.7%, T3c = 17.9% and T4 = 27.1%.

Q36. Answer A

Q37. Answer F

Q38. Answer C

Q39. Answer D

Q40. Answer C

Between 10% and 15% of renal neoplasms are papillary renal cell carcinomas. Two pathological sub-classifications have been described; Type 1 tumours are often multi-focal and have small cells with scanty cytoplasm, arranged in a single layer on the papillary basement membrane with low nuclear grade; Type 2 tumours have a poor prognosis and appear as eosinophilic cells with a high nuclear grade. Type 1 tumours stain positive for CK7 in 78% of cases whilst 80% of type 2 tumours are negative for CK7 [36].

Clear cell renal cell carcinoma accounts for 80%–90% of renal cancers. Loss of function of the VHL gene had been demonstrated in up to 95% of cases. These tumours are usually solitary but appear multifocally in 4% of cases and bilaterally in 3%. Microscopically CCRCC appear as clear cytoplasm cells due to their high content of glycogen and lipids. The growth pattern may be solid, tubular or cystic. CD10 expression has been observed in 94% of cases and CA9 in 90% of clear cell tumours.

Chromophobe RCC accounts for approximately 5% of renal tumours. These tumours appear as large polygonal cells with a transparent slightly reticulated cytoplasm and a prominent cell membrane. Chromophobe RCCs, and in particular the eosinophilic variant, are difficult to distinguish histologically from renal oncocytomas. Hale's colloidal iron stain shows strong reticular pattern in almost 100% of chromophobe RCC.

Collecting duct RCCs are rare tumours that comprise 0.4%–1.8% of all RCCs. Renal medullary carcinoma (RMC) is almost exclusively seen in patients with sickle cell disease or trait. CDCs have a tubulo-papillary architecture that consists of dilated tubules and papillary structures lined by a single layer of cuboidal cells. CDC characteristically co-express low- and high-molecular-weight cytokeratins and react positively to *Ulex europaeus*.

Q41. Answer C

Q42. Answer C

Q43. Answer D

Q44. Answer E

Q45. Answer F

The EAU and AUA guidelines currently recommend partial nephrectomy as the standard of care for the management of T1a small renal masses in patients who are fit for surgery. Several studies have shown that partial nephrectomy offers equivalent oncologic efficacy compared to radical nephrectomy for the treatment of both T1a and T1b renal masses.

The risk of developing a post op eGFR <60 mL/min per 1.73 m^2 following a partial nephrectomy for a T1a SRM in the presence of a normal pre-operative serum creatinine levels and two normal kidneys is 80%, by comparison the risk following a radical nephrectomy is 65% [37]. There is some evidence to suggest that the preservation of renal function associated with partial nephrectomy may have overall health benefits resulting in improved overall survival compared to radical nephrectomy.

The extent of renal injury following hilar vessel clamping during a partial nephrectomy is to a great extent dependent upon the duration of ischaemia time. A recent multicentre series of OPN in solitary kidneys demonstrated that a warm ischaemia time over 20 minutes and a cold ischaemia time greater than 35 minutes was associated with an increased risk of chronic renal insufficiency and acute renal failure [38].

A meta-analysis on the treatment of T1 renal masses performed by the AUA demonstrated that open partial nephrectomy was associated with a 6.3% rate of major urological complications (urine leak, haemorrhage). By comparison laparoscopic partial nephrectomy was associated with a 9.0% incidence of major urological complications [10].

The incidence of positive surgical margins following partial nephrectomy varies between 0% and 10%. The risk of local tumour recurrence subsequent to positive surgical margins varies between 4% and 11%. A recent multicentre study showed that patients with positive surgical margins had similar cancer specific survival and overall survival rates compared to patients with negative surgical margins.

REFERENCES

1. Ljungberg B, Campbell SC, Cho HY, Jacqmin D, Lee JE, Weikert S, et al. The epidemiology of renal cell carcinoma. *Eur Urol.* 2011; 60(4): 615–621.
2. Renehan AG, Tyson M, Egger M, Heller RF, Zwahlen M. Body-mass index and incidence of cancer: A systematic review and meta-analysis of prospective observational studies. *Lancet.* 2008; 371(9612): 569–578.
3. Kutikov A, Uzzo RG. The RENAL nephrometry score: A comprehensive standardized system for quantitating renal tumour size, location and depth. *J Uro.* 2009; 182(3): 844–853.
4. Ficarra V, Novara G, Secco S, Macchi V, Porzionato A, De Caro R, et al. Preoperative aspects and dimensions used for an anatomical (PADUA) classification of renal tumours in patients who are candidates for nephron-sparing surgery. *Eur Urol.* 2009; 56(5): 786–793.
5. Linehan WM, Srinivasan R, Schmidt LS. The genetic basis of kidney cancer: A metabolic disease. *Nat Rev Urol.* 2010; 7(5): 277–285.

6. Kunkle DA, Egleston BL, Uzzo RG. Excise, ablate or observe: The small renal mass dilemma—A meta-analysis and review. *J Urol.* 2008; 179(4): 1227–1233; discussion 1233–1234.

7. Smaldone MC, Kutikov A, Egleston BL, Canter DJ, Viterbo R, Chen DYT, et al. Small renal masses progressing to metastases under active surveillance: A systematic review and pooled analysis. *Cancer.* 2011; 118(4): 997–1006.

8. Edge S, Byrd D, Compton C, Fritz A. *AJCC Cancer Staging Manual.* 7th edn. American Joint Committee on Cancer. Springer, New York, 2010.

9. Capitanio U, Becker F, Blute ML, Mulders P, Patard JJ, Russo P, et al. Lymph node dissection in renal cell carcinoma. *Eur Urol.* 2011; 60(6): 1212–1220.

10. Campbell SC, Novick AC, Belldegrun A, Blute ML, Chow GK, Derweesh IH, et al. Guideline for management of the clinical T1 renal mass. *J Urol.* 2009; 182(4): 1271–1279.

11. Van Poppel H, Becker F, Cadeddu JA, Gill IS, Janetschek G, Jewett MAS, et al. Treatment of localised renal cell carcinoma. *Eur Urol.* 2011; 60(4): 662–672.

12. Phé V, Yates DR, Renard-Penna R, Cussenot O, Roupret M. Is there a contemporary role for percutaneous needle biopsy in the era of small renal masses? *BJU Int.* 2012; 109(6): 867–872.

13. Leveridge MJ, Finelli A, Kachura JR, Evans A, Chung H, Shiff DA, et al. Outcomes of small renal mass needle core biopsy, nondiagnostic percutaneous biopsy, and the role of repeat biopsy. *Eur Urol.* 2011; 60(3): 578–584.

14. Desai MM, Strzempkowski B, Matin SF, Steinberg AP, Ng C, Meraney AM, et al. Prospective randomized comparison of transperitoneal versus retroperitoneal laparoscopic radical nephrectomy. *J Uro.* 2005; 173(1): 38–41.

15. Patard JJ, Pignot G, Escudier B, Eisen T, Bex A, Sternberg C, et al. ICUD-EAU international consultation on kidney cancer 2010: Treatment of metastatic disease. *Eur Urol.* 2011; 60(4): 684–690.

16. Margulis V, McDonald M, Tamboli P, Swanson DA, Wood CG. Predictors of oncological outcome after resection of locally recurrent renal cell carcinoma. *J Urol.* 2009; 181(5): 2044–2051.

17. Frank I, Blute ML, Cheville JC, Lohse CM, Weaver AL, Zincke H. An outcome prediction model for patients with clear cell renal cell carcinoma treated with radical nephrectomy based on tumour stage, size, grade and necrosis: The SSIGN score. *J Urol.* 2002; 168(6): 2395–2400.

18. Sun M, Shariat SF, Cheng C, Ficarra V, Murai M, Oudard S, et al. Prognostic factors and predictive models in renal cell carcinoma: A contemporary review. *Eur Uro.* 2011; 60(4): 644–661.

19. Pea M, Bonetti F, Zamboni G, Martignoni G, Riva M, Colombari R, et al. Melanocyte-marker-HMB-45 is regularly expressed in angiomyolipoma of the kidney. *Pathology.* 1991; 23(3): 185–188.

20. Hora M, Hes O, Reischig T, Urge T, Klecka J, Ferda J, et al. Tumours in end-stage kidney. *Transplant Proc.* 2008; 40(10): 3354–3358.

21. Neuzillet Y, Tillou X, Mathieu R, Long JA, Gigante M, Paparel P, et al. Renal cell carcinoma (RCC) in patients with end-stage renal disease exhibits many favourable clinical, pathologic, and outcome features compared with RCC in the general population. *Eur Urol.* 2011; 60(2): 366–373.

22. Nguyen MM, Gill IS. Effect of renal cancer size on the prevalence of metastasis at diagnosis and mortality. *J Urol.* 2009; 181(3): 1020–1027.

23. Nelson CP, Sanda MG. Contemporary diagnosis and management of renal angiomyolipoma. *J Urol.* 2002; 168(4 Pt 1): 1315–1325.

24. Ouzaid I, Autorino R, Fatica R, Herts BR, McLennan G, Remer EM, et al. Active surveillance for renal angiomyolipoma: Outcomes and factors predictive of delayed intervention. *BJU Int.* 2014 114(3): 412–417.

25. Warren KS, McFarlane J. The Bosniak classification of renal cystic masses. *BJU Int.* 2005; 95(7): 939–942.

26. Bosniak MA. The use of the Bosniak classification system for renal cysts and cystic tumours. *J Urol.* 1997; 157(5): 1852–1853.

27. Bruno JJ, Snyder ME, Motzer RJ, Russo P. Renal cell carcinoma local recurrences, impact of surgical treatment and concomitant metastasis on survival. *BJU Int.* 2006; 97(5): 933–938.

28. Sandhu SS, Symes A, A'Hern R, Sohaib SA, Eisen T, Gore M, et al. Surgical excision of isolated renal-bed recurrence after radical nephrectomy for renal cell carcinoma. *BJU Int.* 2005; 95(4): 522–525.

29. Bani-Hani AH, Leibovich BC, Lohse CM, Cheville JC, Zincke H, Blute ML. Associations with contralateral recurrence following nephrectomy for renal cell carcinoma using a cohort of 2,352 patients. *J Urol.* 2005; 173(2): 391–394.

30. Chapman D, Moore R, Klarenbach S, Braam B. Residual renal function after partial or radical nephrectomy for renal cell carcinoma. *Can Urol Assoc J.* 2010; 4(5): 337–343.

31. Martín OD, Bravo H, Arias M, Dallos D, Quiroz Y, Medina LG, et al. Determinant factors for chronic kidney disease after partial nephrectomy. *Oncoscience.* 2018; 5(1–2): 13–20.

32. Verine J, Pluvinage A, Bousquet G, Lehmann-Che J, de Bazelaire C, Soufir N, et al. Hereditary renal cancer syndromes: An update of a systematic review. *Eur Urol.* 2010; 58: 701–710.

33. Roupret M, Azzouzi A-R, Cussenot O. Microsatellite instability and transitional cell carcinoma of the upper urinary tract. *BJU Int.* 2005; 96(4): 489–492.

34. Di Lorenzo G, Autorino R, Sternberg CN. Metastatic renal cell carcinoma: Recent advances in the targeted therapy era. *Eur Urol.* 2009; 56(6): 959–971.

35. Novara G, Ficarra V, Antonelli A, Artibani W, Bertini R, Carini M, et al. Validation of the 2009 TNM version in a large multi-institutional cohort of patients treated for renal cell carcinoma: Are further improvements needed? *Eur Urol.* 2010; 58(4): 588–595.

36. Algaba F, Akaza H, Lopez-Beltran A, Martignoni G, Moch H, Montironi R, et al. Current pathology keys of renal cell carcinoma. *Eur Urol.* 2011; 60(4): 634–643.

37. Huang WC, Levey AS, Serio AM, Snyder M, Vickers AJ, Raj GV, et al. Chronic kidney disease after nephrectomy in patients with renal cortical tumours: A retrospective cohort study. *Lancet Oncol.* 2006; 7(9): 735–740.

38. Thompson RH, Frank I, Lohse CM, Saad IR, Fergany A, Zincke H, et al. The impact of ischemia time during open nephron sparing surgery on solitary kidneys: A multi-institutional study. *J Urol.* 2007; 177(2): 471–476.

CHAPTER 9: TESTICULAR CANCER

Nkwam Nkwam, Chitranjan J. Shukla, David A. Manson-Bahr, Taimur T. Shah and Farooq Khan

MCQs

Q1. Regarding orchidectomy for testicular cancer, which of the following is TRUE?
- A. Testicular prosthesis can be inserted without fear of prohibitive infectious complications.
- B. Division of the spermatic cord must be taken at the superficial inguinal ring.
- C. In cases of symptomatic metastatic disease orchidectomy should precede chemotherapy.
- D. Organ-sparing surgery can be performed when tumour volume is less than 50%.
- E. Long-term risk of silicone implants is well known.

Q2. Regarding testicular cancer, which of the following is TRUE?
- A. Incidence is 2 per 100,000 males in Western countries.
- B. 3%–5% are bilateral at diagnosis.
- C. Magnetic resonance imaging is the imaging of choice for diagnosis.
- D. Magnetic resonance imaging is more sensitive than ultrasound for diagnosis.
- E. Tumour markers provide no prognostic information.

Q3. In the staging & diagnosis of testicular cancer, which of the following is TRUE?
- A. CT thorax, abdomen & pelvis is recommended in all patients.
- B. Discuss sperm banking in all men after orchidectomy.
- C. Five-year survival for 'good prognosis' seminoma is 96%.
- D. In the TNM staging classification pN2 means a lymph node mass >5 cm.
- E. In the TNM staging classification M1b means non-regional lymph node(s) or lung metastasis.

Q4. Regarding tumour markers in testicular cancer, which of the following is TRUE?
- A. HCG has a half-life of 5–7 days.
- B. AFP has a half-life of 48–72 hours.
- C. In non-seminomatous germ cell tumours an HCG of 5,000 confers poor prognosis.
- D. Pure seminomas never secrete AFP.
- E. In seminomas an HCG >50,000 confers poor prognosis.

Q5. Regarding germ cell neoplasia in situ (GCNIS), which of the following is TRUE?
- A. Overall incidence in the contralateral testis is approximately 10%.
- B. Incidence of a contralateral metachronous tumour is approximately 10%.
- C. Biopsy of the contralateral testis is mandatory in most cases.
- D. Chemotherapy is more effective than radiotherapy in its treatment.
- E. Five-year risk of developing testicular cancer is 90% with a normal contralateral testis.

Q6. Regarding the epidemiology of testis cancer, which of the following is FALSE?
- A. The trend for incidence has been one of decline.
- B. Sweden has a higher incidence than Finland.

C. Within the UK, the average incidence is highest in Scotland.

D. Germ cell tumours account for 95% of testis tumours.

E. Cryptorchidism increases the risk of testicular cancer in the undescended testis as well as the contralateral descended testis.

Q7. **With regards to germ cell neoplasia in situ (GCNIS) of the testis, which of the following is TRUE?**

A. The incidence is approximately 5%.

B. The progression rate to carcinoma is approximately 15% over 5 years.

C. Testicular microlithiasis is an independent risk factor.

D. If diagnosed on biopsy of remaining testis post-orchidectomy for testis cancer, the mainstay of treatment would currently involve radiotherapy, which does not impact on endocrine function.

E. If diagnosed on biopsy of remaining testis post-orchidectomy for testis cancer, the mainstay of treatment would currently involve radiotherapy, which does not impact on fertility.

Q8. **Which of the following is FALSE with regard to tumour markers in testis cancer?**

A. The half-life of Alpha-fetoprotein (AFP) is 24–36 hours.

B. Of all patients with testis cancer approximately half have a raised tumour marker reading.

C. Lactate dehydrogenase is a ubiquitous enzyme which is non-specific for tumour type.

D. A very high level of βHCG may suggest a seminoma with syncytiotrophoblastic cells.

E. They may be elevated in up to 90% of non-seminomatous germ cell tumours.

Q9. **Which of the following does NOT cause serum HCG to rise?**

A. Hydatidiform mole

B. Marijuana use

C. Testicular lymphoma

D. Hypogonadism

E. Testicular seminoma

Q10. **With regards to the genetics of testis cancer, which of the following is TRUE?**

A. The gene locus for testis cancer is likely to be at Xq27.

B. The risk is higher if the father is affected than if a sibling is affected.

C. The gene locus for testis cancer is likely to be at 12q27.

D. Inheritance is in a Mendelian fashion as autosomal recessive.

E. None of the above.

Q11. **With regards to testis preserving surgery in testis cancer, which of the following is FALSE?**

A. Indications include bilateral tumours, tumour in a solitary testis, non-palpable tumour.

B. It should be attempted for benign lesions.

C. It should be performed in high-volume centralised units.

D. The tumour must be polar and occupy <50% of the volume of the testis.

E. Can be performed via an inguinal approach using a Chevassu procedure.

Q12. **Which of the following is NOT an adverse prognostic marker in stage I non-seminomatous germ cell tumour?**

A. Vascular invasion

B. Tumour size

C. Proliferation rate >70%

D. Percentage of embryonal carcinoma in >50%

E. Absence of teratoma

Q13. **With regards to risk stratification in germ cell tumours, which of the following is FALSE?**

A. Occult metastasis rate for a patient with a 5 cm seminoma not affecting the rete testis is approximately 15%.

B. Occult metastasis rate for a patient with a 2 cm seminoma not affecting the rete testis is approximately 6%.

C. Occult metastasis rate for a patient with a NSGCT without vascular invasion is approximately 20%.

D. Occult metastasis rate for a patient with a NSGCT with vascular invasion is approximately 50%.

E. Occult metastasis rate for a patient with a 6 cm seminoma affecting the rete testis is approximately 30%.

Q14. Regarding the histology of non-seminomatous germ cell tumours, which of the following is associated with an increased risk of metastasis in cases apparently stage 1 at presentation?
A. Positive staining for AFP
B. Lymphovascular invasion
C. Presence of undifferentiated cells
D. Absence of yolk sac elements
E. Cord invasion

Q15. Which of the following is TRUE of metastatic seminoma?
A. A raised serum AFP is most unusual.
B. Lung metastases frequently occur in the absence of lymph node metastases.
C. Back pain is a common symptom.
D. A raised serum HCG is rarely seen.
E. There will always be a previous history of testicular tumour.

Q16. GCNIS of the contralateral testis in a patient with testicular tumour is associated with an incidence of subsequent tumour development at 5 years out:
A. 20%
B. 35%
C. 50%
D. 75%
E. 9%

Q17. Which of the following is associated with an increased incidence of carcinoma in situ of the testis (germ cell neoplasia in situ [GCNIS])?
A. Kartagener's syndrome
B. Diabetes mellitus
C. Solvent abuse
D. Some intersex syndromes
E. Bilateral cryptorchidism

Q18. Which of the following is TRUE regarding alpha-fetoprotein (AFP)?
A. Is produced by pure seminomatous germ cell tumours
B. Is produced by pure choriocarcinoma
C. Is produced by both seminomatous and non-seminomatous germ cell tumours
D. Is only produced by germ cell tumours
E. Is the foetal homologue of serum albumin

Q19. Which of the following is FALSE regarding human chorionic gonadotrophin (HCG)?
A. Is produced by the human placenta
B. Is also known as β-HCG
C. Is only produced by germ cell tumours
D. Is always produced by gestational trophoblastic disease
E. Is particularly useful in monitoring seminomatous germ cell tumours

Q20. Which of the following is TRUE regarding oligospermia following successful treatment of a non-seminomatous testicular tumour?
A. May persist more than 1 year after orchidectomy
B. Is best prevented by LHRH analogues in case of chemotherapy
C. Is very rare at the time of diagnosis of non-seminomatous germ cell tumour (NSGCT)
D. Is present in 50% of patients following modified bilateral template retroperitoneal lymph node dissection
E. Is completely reversible after 18 months

Q21. A patient with a non-seminomatous germ cell testicular tumour has normal CT of the chest, abdomen and pelvis. HCG and AFP persist at a high level after orchidectomy. What is the best strategy?
A. Chemotherapy
B. Radical lymph node dissection
C. Surveillance until metastases become apparent
D. Modified nerve sparing lymph node dissection
E. Repeat tumour markers after an interval of 6 months

Q22. In cases where a NSGCT has rising tumour markers after orchidectomy and a normal staging CT scan the next step should be?
A. FDG-PET CT scan
B. Choline PET CT scan

C. Ultrasound scan of contralateral testis
D. Chemotherapy
E. Retroperitoneal lymph node dissection

EMQs

Each answer can be used more than once

Q23–28. Regarding staging for patients with testicular cancer
A. Embryonal carcinoma <50%
B. Embryonal carcinoma >50%
C. Proliferation rate >50%
D. Proliferation rate >70%
E. Rete testis invasion
F. Tumour size >3 cm
G. Tumour size >4 cm
H. pT1
I. pT2
J. pT3
K. pT4
L. pN1
M. pN2
N. pN3
O. M1a
P. M1b

Q23. Risk factors for metastatic disease in stage 1 seminoma? (select two answers).

Q24. Risk factors for metastatic disease in stage 1 non-seminomatous germ cell tumours? (select two answers).

Q25. In the TNM classification multiple lymph node metastases <2 cm in diameter is staged as? (select one answer).

Q26. In the TNM classification non-regional lymph node(s) involvement is staged as? (select one answer).

Q27. In the TNM classification (2017) tumour limited to the testis with lymphovascular invasion is staged as? (select one answer).

Q28. In the TNM classification (2017) tumour that invades the scrotal wall without lymphovascular invasion is staged as? (select one answer).

Q29–35. Regarding relapse in patients with testicular cancer
A. 5%
B. 6%
C. 12%
D. 15%
E. 30%
F. 32%
G. 50%
H. 99%
I. AUO trial AH 01/94
J. Medical Research Council Report 1996
K. MRC TE18
L. MRC TE19
M. SWENOTWECA

Q29. Sensitivity of ultrasound in the diagnosis of testicular cancer? (select one answer).

Q30. Absence of two risk factors for stage 1 seminoma for confers a retroperitoneal relapse rate of? (select one answer).

Q31. The presence of two risk factors for stage 1 seminoma confers a retroperitoneal relapse rate of? (select one answer).

Q32. A single dose of carboplatin in stage 1 seminoma reduces relapse rate at 5 years to? (select one answer).

Q33. This study compared the use of 30 Gy versus 20 Gy in the adjuvant treatment of stage I testicular seminoma? (select one answer).

Q34. This study demonstrated a 90% relative risk reduction in relapse rates of stage 1 NSGCT with single-course bleomycin, etoposide, cisplatin (BEP) chemotherapy? (select one answer).

Q35. Overall relapse rate of stage 1 NSCGT? (select one answer).

Q36–40. Regarding chemotherapeutic agents for testicular cancer
   A. Bleomycin
   B. eGFR < 60
   C. Cisplatin
   D. Etoposide
   E. Glove and stocking peripheral neuropathy
   F. Liver cirrhosis
   G. Nephrotoxicity
   H. Neuropathy with acute pain
   I. Paclitaxel
   J. Pulmonary pneumonitis and fibrosis
   K. Radiotherapy
   L. Smokers
   M. Vinblastine

Q36. Common side effect of Bleomycin?

Q37. Group of patients in whom Bleomycin is contraindicated?

Q38. Patient presents with tinnitus may have received this agent?

Q39. Patient presents with a painful neuropathy may have received this agent?

Q40. Cisplatin is contraindicated in these patients?

Q41–44. Staging of testicular cancer using the TNM staging system
   A. pT1N2M0S0
   B. pT1N1M0S0
   C. pT2N2M0S1
   D. pT3N3M1aS2

E. pTXN3M1bS2
F. pTXN3M1bS3
G. pTXN3M1aS3
H. pT2N1M0S0
I. pT2N2M0S0

Q41. A patient underwent left orchidectomy, the specimen showed a seminoma with rete testis invasion, but no invasion of tunica and cord structures. CT showed a single node of 1.5 cm in the para-aortic region. Tumour markers were normal. What is the correct staging category?

Q42. A patient presents breathless with a large solid left testicular mass extending up the scrotal neck but not involving the scrotal skin. Tumour marker readings were AFP 2 ng/mL, βHCG 7,200 mIU/mL, LDH 1,000 u/L (normal up to 250 u/L) and CT showed extensive nodal masses including one at the left renal hilum (5 cm) causing hydronephrosis and lung metastases. What is the correct staging category?

Q43. A 35-year-old man with an extra-gonadal tumour, arising from the pelvis with extensive intra-abdominal metastases to nodes, liver, lung and tumour markers with AFP of 12,000 ng/mL, βHCG 64,200 mIU/mL and LDH of 12,000 u/L. What is the correct staging category?

Q44. A 27-year-old man underwent orchidectomy, the specimen showing a NSGCT with lymphatic invasion, but no invasion of tunica vaginalis and cord structures. CT showed 2 nodes node of 1.5 cm each in the para-aortic region. Tumour markers were AFP 2 ng/mL, βHCG 7.2 mIU/mL, LDH 100 u/L. What is the correct staging category?

Q45–47. Regarding treatment of testis cancer after orchidectomy
   A. Retroperitoneal lymph node dissection
   B. Laparoscopic retroperitoneal lymph node biopsy

C. Carboplatin

D. Bleomycin, etoposide and cisplatin (BEP) courses

E. Dog-leg radiotherapy

F. Full template radiotherapy

G. Second line chemotherapy

H. Surveillance

I. Second line/salvage chemotherapy

J. None

Q45. A 45-year-old man post-orchidectomy with normal pre-op CT and tumour markers. His histology of the testis confirmed a classical seminoma of 5 cm with rete testis invasion. What would the treatment of choice be?

Q46. A 75-year-old man post-orchidectomy who had an HCG of 5, normal other markers and whose CT was normal pre-operatively. His histology of the testis confirmed a spermatocytic seminoma. What would the treatment of choice be?

Q47. A 25-year-old man in the UK who had an orchidectomy for stage I NSGCT and had a para-aortic node of 1.5 cm. What would the treatment of choice be?

MCQs – ANSWERS

Q1. Answer A

From a large series of testicular prosthesis insertions at radical inguinal orchidectomy (Robinson et al., BJUI 2016) 33 of 885 patients were re-admitted with a variety of post-op complications including infection within 30 days. However, only 1 out of 236 patients (0.4%) required prosthesis removal.

The spermatic cord is tied and excised at the deep inguinal ring.

Symptomatic metastatic disease is an oncological emergency and first line treatment should be expedited chemotherapy.

The guidelines for organ-sparing surgery involve the tumour volume to be less than 30%.

The long-term risks of silicone implants remain unknown despite the controversy with breast implants.

Q2. Answer D

The incidence of testicular cancer is 10 per 100,000 and 1%–2% are bilateral.

Although ultrasound (US) of the testes has a sensitivity of almost 100% MRI is still more sensitive and specific but its cost-effectiveness over US is not justifiable.

The IGCCCT (International Germ Cell Cancer Collaborative) prognostic-based staging system utilises AFP, HCG and LDH to determine different prognostic groups for metastatic tumours and the TNM classification uses tumour markers for their staging S groups.

Q3. Answer A

Sperm banking must be discussed in all men before orchidectomy and chemotherapy in cases of delayed orchidectomy due to a significant number of these patients have poor quality semen analysis across the board preoperatively. The five-year survival for good prognosis classical seminoma is 86%. M1a is correct answer as M1b is distant metastases other than non-regional lymph nodes such as brain metastases.

Q4. Answer D

HCG has a half-life is 48–72 hours whereas AFP has a half-life of 3–5 days. HCG level of 5,000–50,000 confers intermediate prognosis in the IGCCCT prognostic grouping and there is no poor prognosis group for pure seminomas.

Q5. Answer A

Overall incidence of GCNIS in the contralateral testis is approximately 10% with a 50% five-year risk of developing testicular cancer. Incidence of a contralateral metachronous tumour is approximately with current EAU guidelines identified risk factors for detecting GCNIS which is the reason to biopsy the contralateral testis and found that patients presenting younger than 31 years of age, and those with a small testis (<12 mL), history of undescended testes, or poor spermatogenesis (Johnsen score of 1–3) had higher rates of GCNIS that could be as high as 34%. Radiotherapy is the treatment of choice for confirmed GCNIS and is given at a dose of 16–20 Gy in fractions of 2 Gy. If patient is undergoing post-orchidectomy chemo, then there is a 66% chance of treating ITGCN, and a rebiopsy after 2 years would be sensible.

Q6. Answer A

The trend of testis cancer is one of increasing incidence, the reason not being clear but dietary and environmental factors no doubt will be contributing to this. Rising incidence is seen with geographical increasing latitudes with Scotland having the highest incidence in the UK.

Although you may not be expected to know all the intricacies of the epidemiology of individual European nations, it is relevant to know that the trend is on the increase.

Q7. Answer D

The incidence across the general population is 0.8%. The incidence of GCNIS in the contralateral testis in patient with a testicular cancer is 5%. Progression to carcinoma is 50% at 5 years and 70% at 7 years. Testicular microlithiasis is not an independent risk factor and as per EAU guidelines and is only relevant in patients with other risk factors (such as cryptorchidism or atrophy) and exists in 2%–6% of the general population. Once GCNIS is diagnosed in the remaining testis, radiotherapy is advised which will affect spermatogonia and render patients subfertile but will not affect Leydig cell function.

Q8. Answer A

AFP has a half-life of 5–7 days. β hCG has a half-life of 24–36 hours. These need to be borne in mind when checking post-operative or post-treatment levels. Lactate dehydrogenase (LDH) is a ubiquitous enzyme which is non-specific for tumour type. Overall 50% of patients will have raised markers at diagnosis. 5%–10% of pure seminomas will have a raised β hCG (produced by syncytiotrophoblast elements). 90% of non-seminomatous GCTs may have elevated markers. 50%–70% will have a raised AFP (produced by yolk sac elements) and 40% will have a raised β hCG. β hCG is raised in 100% of choriocarcinoma's and 40%–60% of embryonal carcinoma.

Q9. Answer C

All except testicular lymphoma can cause a rise in HCG to some degree.

Q10. Answer A

The risk is higher if a sibling is affected meaning that the gene locus is likely to be on the X chromosome. Familial studies have suggested a LOD (Logarithm of Odds) in the region of 2 (i.e., suggestive but not definitive of a familial inheritance pattern).

Q11. Answer D

Tumour volume should be <30%. Indications are A & B. As these are uncommonly indicated, they should be performed in high-volume centres with expertise to use intra-operative ultrasound localisation or by bi-valving the testis after soft clamps are used to occlude the blood supply (the Chevassu procedure).

Q12. Answer B

Vascular/lymphatic invasion, proliferation rate >70% and percentage of embryonal carcinoma >50% are all prognostic markers for occult metastatic disease in non-seminoma stage I. Absence of teratoma can also independently complement vascular invasion.

Tumour size (>4 cm) is an adverse prognostic marker for stage I seminoma along with rete testis invasion.

Q13. Answer B

Risk stratification is evidence-based. In NSGCT tumours with low risk disease (i.e., without vascular/lymphatic invasion), recurrence rate is approximately 20% compared to 50% for high risk disease (with vascular/lymphatic invasion) and an overall rate of 30% (Read et al. *Journal of Clinical Oncology* 1992 and Albers et al. *Journal of Clinical Oncology* 2003). In seminomatous tumours, low-risk disease (i.e., no adverse features like rete testis invasion and tumour <4 cm), recurrence is 12%, and if one risk factor is present, it is approximately 16%, and if both are present, it is 32%, giving an overall recurrence rate of 20%. It is important to note that whilst we all use these features, this is from a large retrospective series and has not been shown prospectively. The data from the TRISST study will help with this. Single-dose carboplatin chemotherapy or traditional 'dog-leg' radiotherapy reduces the risk recurrence to approximately 4% in seminoma.

Q14. Answer B

The key histological parameter in determining risk of occult metastatic disease in NSGCT is lymphovascular invasion (LVI) with 48% developing metastases in LVI is present compared to 14% for those without LVI.

Q15. Answer A

Pure seminoma's and choriocarcinoma do not produce AFP.

Q16. Answer C

There is a 10% risk of contralateral germ cell neoplasia in situ (GCNIS) with 50% developing into testicular cancer within 5-years. Those who are less than 40 years of ago with a testicular volume of less than 12cc have a 34% risk of GCNIS and should undergo contralateral biopsy (EAU guidelines). Two biopsies should be taken from the upper and lower pole. There is also an increased risk in those with undescended tests and subfertility.

Q17. Answer E

Risk factors for contralateral tumour or GCNIS include a history of previous testicular cancer, infertility, undescended testis, Klinefelter syndrome and family history of testicular cancer in a first-degree relative.

Q18. Answer E

In addition to GCT of the testes raised AFP levels can be seen in patients with liver cancer or less commonly other cancers (for stomach, bowel, lung, breast and lymphoma). Mildly raised levels are also seen with chronic hepatitis or cirrhosis.

Q19. Answer C

HCG may be raised in seminomatous and non-seminomatous testicular germ cell tumours as well as a hydatidiform moles and choriocarcinoma in women. Other tumours may lead to mildly raised HCG levels, and these include hepatic and pancreatic neuroendocrine tumours.

Q20. Answer A

Weak or absent ejaculation is present in 50% of patients following modified retroperitoneal lymph node dissection. Oligospermia can persist for some time following treatment of testis cancer, even following orchidectomy and separate to the effects of chemotherapy, and hence, the need to sperm bank preoperatively.

Q21. Answer A

The correct answer is A, as no lymph nodes are seen on CT. If the marker level for AFP or HCG increases after orchidectomy, the patient has residual disease. An US examination of the contralateral testicle must be performed. In case of NSGCT, if RPLND is performed, up to 87% of these patients have pathologically documented nodes in the retroperitoneum. The treatment of true Clinical Stage 1S NSGT patients is still controversial. They may be treated with chemotherapy and with follow-up as for Clinical Stage 1B patients (high risk, see below) after primary chemotherapy or by RPLND. In the UK and Europe standard practice is chemotherapy then RPLND if required. Primary RPLND is reserved for those with retroperitoneal (RP) mass, normal tumour markers and TD in the primary and it is felt that the RP nodes are only TD. TD may appear cystic on imaging.

Q22. Answer C

FDG-PET CT is the most commonly used PET scan in patients with testicular cancer. Its role is limited to patients with seminoma and a residual retroperitoneal mass greater than 3 cm.

EMQs – ANSWERS

Q23. Answers G and E

Q24. Answers B and D

Q25. Answer L

Q26. Answer O

Q27. Answer I

Q28. Answer K

TNM classification for testicular cancer (2017)

pTX	Primary tumour cannot be assessed
pT0	No evidence of primary tumour (e.g. histological scar in testis)
pTis	Intratubular germ cell neoplasia (testicular intraepithelial neoplasia)
pT1	Tumour limited to testis and epididymis without vascular/lymphatic invasion; tumour may invade tunica albuginea but not tunica vaginalis
pT2	Tumour limited to testis and epididymis with vascular/lymphatic invasion, or tumour extending through tunica albuginea with involvement of tunica vaginalis
pT3	Tumour invades spermatic cord with or without vascular/lymphatic invasion
pT4	Tumour invades scrotum with or without vascular/lymphatic invasion
NX	Regional lymph nodes cannot be assessed
N0	No regional lymph node metastasis
N1	Metastasis with a lymph node mass 2 cm or less in greatest dimension or multiple lymph nodes, none more than 2 cm in greatest dimension
N2	Metastasis with a lymph node mass more than 2 cm but not more than 5 cm in greatest dimension, or multiple lymph nodes, any one mass more than 2 cm but not more than 5 cm in greatest dimension
N3	Metastasis with a lymph node mass more than 5 cm in greatest dimension
MX	Distant metastasis cannot be assessed
M0	No distant metastasis
M1	Distant metastasis
M1a	Non-regional lymph node(s) or lung
M1b	Other sites
SX	Serum marker studies not available or not performed
S0	Serum marker study levels within normal limits
S1	LDH up to 1.5× normal; BHCG <5,000, AFP <1,000
S2	In between S1 and S3
S3	LDH up to 10× normal; BHCG >50,000, AFP >10,000

Stage 1 – N0, M0, (5% will be stage 1 marker positive S 1-3, indicating sub clinical metastases)
- 1a – T1
- 1b – T2-4
- 1s – Markers S1 – S3

Stage 2 – N1-3, M0

Stage 3 – N1-3, M1, (S2-3)

Tis   ITGCN

T1   Tunica Albuginea WITHOUT LVI

T2   Tunica Vaginalis or LVI

T3   Spermatic cord

T4   Scrotum

Q29. Answer H

Q30. Answer C

Q31. Answer F

Q32. Answer A

Q33. Answer K

Q34. Answer M

Q35. Answer E

MRC TE19 Trial by Oliver et al. published in *The Lancet* in 2005 (updated in *J Clin Onc*, 2011) was a multicenter multinational (UK & Belgium) randomised trial that compared radiotherapy (RT) to single dose carboplatin in 1,477 men with clinical stage 1 (pT1-pT3, S0) seminoma. Carboplatin was administered at (7x GFR + 25 mg) and RT was delivered using para-aortic/dog-leg at 20–30 Gy. Relapse-free rate was 94.7% versus 96.0%, respectively.

The MRC TE18 study was published by Jones et al. (*J Clin Onc* 2005); it found the absolute difference in 2-year relapse rates to be 0.7%. Treatment with 20 Gy in 10 fractions is unlikely to produce relapse rates more than 3% higher than for standard 30 Gy radiation therapy with lower incidence of lethargy at 4 weeks post-RT compared to 30 Gy.

SWENOTECA by Tornstad et al. published in *J Clin Onc* (2009) was a prospective community-based multicentre Swedish and Norwegian Testicular Cancer Project (SWENOTECA) management programme looking at risk-adapted treatment in clinical stage I NSGCTs. Lymphovascular invasion (LVI) positive patients received BEP chemotherapy and LVI negative patients received BEP or surveillance. In the LVI positive patients who had surveillance or BEP x1 relapse rates were 41% and 3.2%, respectively. Similarly, in the LVI negative cohorts relapse rates for the same were 13% and 1.3%, respectively. Hence, the authors concluded that BEP x1 reduces the risk of relapse by 90% in both LVI positive and LVI negative clinical stage 1 (CS1) NSGCT.

Up to 30% of NSGCT patients with CS1 disease will have occult metastatic disease and relapse during surveillance; 80% of relapses occur during the first 12 months of follow-up, 12% during the second year and 6% during the third year, decreasing to 1% during the fourth and fifth years.

Q36. Answer J

Q37. Answer L

Q38. Answer C

Q39. Answer I

Q40. Answer B

Bleomycin can cause lung pneumonitis and fibrosis and is best avoided in smokers and those over 40 years of age or those with high lung metastases.

Cisplatin can cause a range of side effects. It is nephrotoxic and is contraindicated in patients with an eGFR of <60 mL/min/1.73 m^2. Ototoxicity is another common side effect where patients present with tinnitus and hearing loss. An increased risk of acute myeloid leukaemia has also been observed along with increased risk of hypogonadism and cardiovascular disease.

Secondary solid and haematological malignancies have been reported after both radiotherapy and chemotherapy.

Q41. Answer B

Q42. Answer D

Q43. Answer F

Q44. Answer H

Please see TNM classification above.

Q45. Answer C

Q46. Answer J

Q47. Answer D

For seminoma, the International Germ Cell Cancer Consensus Group (IGCCCG) good metastatic prognostic group include patients with pulmonary Mets and should receive either 3 x BEP or 4 x EP or RT 30 Gy (dog-leg RT if no pulmonary metastases). Intermediate group patients are those with non-pulmonary Mets and should receive 4 x BEP or 4 x PEI (cisplatin, etoposide, ifosfamide). A residual retroperitoneal mass after chemotherapy for seminoma is not usually worrying. If >3 cm a reasonable course of action would be a FDG-PET at 4–6 weeks. If hot on PET then either a biopsy followed by chemotherapy or radiotherapy could be offered. Although RPLND is rarely used in seminoma some advocate its use to reduce the chemotherapy burden on the patient.

Recurrences after stage 1 seminoma should be treated with chemotherapy regimens as for primary metastatic disease. For stage 2 seminoma with a less than 2 cm nodal mass and negative markers, biopsy or surveillance for 8 weeks are both reasonable options. If mass is growing but markers are negative then consider RPLND. If markers are rising then offer chemotherapy. Some centres might perform a RPLND with a single cycle of carboplatin to avoid long-term toxicity of cisplatin.

Non-seminoma (NSGCT) IGCCCG good prognostic group patients can have nodal and pulmonary metastases with S1 markers. They should receive 3 x BEP or 4 x EP. Intermediate prognostic group can have nodal and pulmonary metastases with S2 markers and should receive 4 x BEP or PEI (cisplatin, etoposide, ifosfamide). Poor prognostic group have mediastinal primary or visceral metastases or are maker S3 and should also undergo 4 x BEP or PEI. Salvage chemotherapy (TIP, (cisplatin, ifosfamide, paclitaxel)) should be offered if there is a residual mass at 4–12 weeks and markers are positive. In marker negative disease with a residual mass >1 cm patients should be offered RPLND. There is no role for PET in NSGCT's. At RPLND, 50% will have necrosis, 35% mature teratoma and 15% will have viable cancer. For necrosis or mature teratoma then surveillance is reasonable. If viable tumour is found then further salvage chemotherapy should be offered. Desperation surgery/RPLND can be offered for marker positive disease only after salvage chemotherapy with 20%–50% achieving remission.

CHAPTER 10: PENILE CANCER

Hussain M. Alnajjar and Asif Muneer

MCQs

Q1. Which of the following is NOT a risk factor for penile carcinoma?
A. Smoking
B. Phimosis
C. Chlamydial infection
D. Exposure to ultraviolet light
E. HPV 16 and 18 infection

Q2. Which of these tumour markers is NOT associated with penile squamous cell carcinoma?
A. SCC antigen
B. Ki-67
C. p53
D. HSV-2
E. E-cadherin

Q3. With regards to the mechanism of action of 5 Flurouracil (5–FU) cream for erythroplasia of Queyrat (EQ). Which of the following is TRUE?
A. RNA synthesis is blocked.
B. It alters the host immune system.
C. DNA synthesis is blocked.
D. It inhibits thymidylate reductase.
E. It is an anti-tumour antibiotic.

Q4. What would be the EAU recommended first-line treatment for a man with a biopsy proven SCC on the glans penis that is confined to the corpus spongiosus on staging MRI (cT2 disease)?
A. Partial penectomy
B. Radical radiotherapy
C. Radical penectomy with a perineal urethrostomy
D. Glansectomy with a split-thickness skin graft
E. Total glans resurfacing

Q5. Which of the following is dynamic sentinel lymph node biopsy (DSLNB) for staging in patients with proven SCC of the penis indicated for?
A. Clinically palpable inguinal lymph nodes
B. Fixed recurrent inguinal nodal mass post prior modified inguinal lymphadenectomy
C. Clinically impalpable inguinal lymph nodes
D. Clinically impalpable inguinal lymph nodes with positive fine needle aspiration cytology
E. Contralateral clinically palpable inguinal lymph nodes during inguinal lymphadenectomy for palpable disease

Q6. Which of the following is NOT an anatomical boundary of the femoral triangle?
A. The inguinal ligament
B. Medial border of adductor longus muscle
C. Medial border of sartorius muscle
D. Iliopsoas, pectineus muscles and femoral vessels
E. Lateral border of adductor longus muscle

Q7. Which primary tumour pathological feature is NOT associated with increased risk of lymph node metastases and poorer prognosis?
A. Stage T2 or greater
B. Grade 3/4
C. Basaloid subtype
D. Perineural and vascular invasion
E. Tumour location

Q8. With regards to the EAU guidelines on penile cancer 2013. How frequently should a man be followed up during the first 2 years following penile preserving surgery and a negative sentinel lymph node biopsy?
A. Monthly
B. 2 monthly
C. 3 monthly
D. 4 monthly
E. 6 monthly

Q9. Which of the following is NOT a recognised treatment option for penile intraepithelial neoplasia (PeIN)?
A. Wide local excision (WLE) with circumcision
B. Laser therapy
C. Topical 5 flurouracil (5 FU) or imiquimod
D. Radiotherapy
E. Total glans resurfacing surgery

Q10. Which of the following stages of penile SCC should be recommended adjuvant chemotherapy?
A. pN2 and pN3 disease
B. pN1 disease
C. pT3 N0 disease
D. pT2 N1 disease
E. PeIN

Q11. Which of the following are NOT recognised preventative measures for penile squamous cell carcinoma?
A. Neonatal circumcision
B. Prophylactic HPV vaccination
C. Cessation of smoking
D. Avoiding PUVA treatment
E. Prophylactic HSV vaccination

Q12. Which of the following viruses is consistently found on histological review in up to 50% of specimens and has a causal role in the pathogenesis of penile squamous cell carcinoma?
A. Human papillomavirus (HPV) type 18
B. HPV type 16
C. HPV type 30
D. HPV type 31
E. Herpes simplex virus (HSV)

Q13. Which of the following penile dermatosis is NOT associated with penile cancer?
A. Lichen sclerosus (LS)
B. Bowenoid papulosis
C. Paget's disease
D. Buschke–Löwenstein (Giant condyloma)
E. Condyloma acuminatum

Q14. A 69-year-old man presents to your clinic with the following lesion on his glans and inner prepuce. The lesion persists despite topical steroid and antifungal creams. A biopsy is obtained and reveals undifferentiated PeIN. What is this lesion known as?

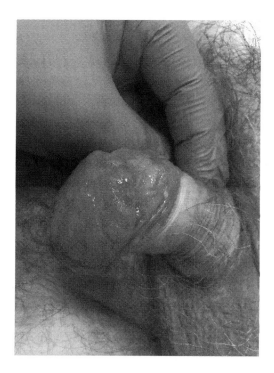

A. Bowen disease
B. Bowenoid papulosis
C. Erythroplasia of Queyrat
D. Buschke–Löwenstein (giant condyloma)
E. Paget's disease

EMQs

Q15-17. AJCC 2017 TNM 8th Edition staging system for penile cancer
A. Tis
B. Ta
C. T1aN0M0
D. T1bN0M0
E. T2N1M0
F. T2N3M0
G. T3N1M0
H. T3N2M0
I. T4N3M1

For each of the following clinical statements, choose the correct TNM classification from the list above.

Q15. Which of the above stages is correct for a non-invasive verrucous carcinoma?

Q16. Which of the above is the correct stage for a tumour invading the corpus spongiosum with metastasis in a single inguinal lymph node?

Q17. Which of the above is the correct stage when the tumour invades lamina propria and is poorly differentiated (Grade 3 or 4), with negative DSLNB and no metastases?

Q18-20. Diagnosis and staging investigations of a suspicious penile mass
A. Ultrasound and fine needle aspiration cytology (USS + FNAC)
B. Urine microscopy, culture and sensitivity
C. CT chest/abdomen and pelvis
D. MRI penis with alprostadil injection
E. DSLNB
F. Penile biopsy
G. DSLNB following a negative USS+ FNAC
H. CT/PET
I. Modified bilateral inguinal lymph node dissections

For each of the scenarios below, choose the correct next investigation from the list above.

Q18. Investigation required prior to definitive surgery of a suspicious penile mass after physical examination?

Q19. The next investigation for a man with a pT1b G3 SCC of the penis and impalpable inguinal lymph nodes?

Q20. The investigation that has been found to improve local staging of a penile mass?

Q21-24. Treatment options for the primary lesion in a man with a biopsy proven SCC of the penis
A. Radical penectomy and perineal urethrostomy formation
B. Partial penectomy
C. Circumcision
D. Wide local excision
E. Topical 5-fluorouracil (5-FU) cream
F. Glansectomy and split skin graft reconstruction
G. Total glans resurfacing
H. Glansectomy + distal corporectomy and split-thickness skin graft repair

For each of the following clinical scenarios below, what would be the preferred treatment option, from the list above?

Q21. Preputial pTa tumour.

Q22. Frail 85-year-old man with a large fungating tumour (cT3/4).

Q23. Previously circumcised 35-year-old man with widespread erythroplasia of Queyrat refractory to topical therapy?

Q24. Biopsy confirmed undifferentiated PeIN measuring 0.5 cm in diameter on dorsum of the glans penis.

Q25-27. Histology of carcinoma of the penis
A. Squamous cell carcinoma (SCC)
B. Extramammary Paget's disease
C. Malignant melanoma
D. Basal cell carcinoma
E. Basaloid subtype of SCC
F. Verrucous subtype of SCC
G. Usual (classic) subtype of SCC

For each of the following statements below, what would be the preferred histological scenario, from the list above?

Q25. Accounts for 95% of all malignant penile disease

Q26. Aggressive subtype with a poorer prognosis

Q27. Accounts for approximately 60%–70% of SCCs

Q28–30. Epidemiology of penile carcinoma
    A. 0.1–0.9 per 100,000 men/year
    B. 4.4 per 100,000 men/year
    C. 20 per 100,000 men/year
    D. 0.1–0.9 per 10,000 men/year
    E. 100 cases new per year

    F. 400 cases new per year
    G. 5000 cases new per year

For each of the following statements below, what would be the correct epidemiological description, from the list above?

Q28. The incidence of penile cancer in the UK and Europe

Q29. The incidence of penile cancer in Uganda

Q30. The approximate number of new penile cancer cases in the UK per annum

MCQs – ANSWERS

Q1. Answer C

All the above except chlamydial infection predisposes to SCC of the penis. BXO or lichen sclerosus et atrophicus is now also believed to be a risk factor.

Q2. Answer D

Herpes Simplex Virus-2 (HSV-2) is a sexually transmitted chronic infection of the genital tract and is not a biomarker for SCC of the penis. Other markers associated with penile SCC include p16INK4A, MMP-2, HPV DNA, PTEN, HER3/4 and miRNA.

Q3. Answer C

Topical 5 FU is structurally similar to thymine and blocks DNA synthesis by inhibiting thymidylate synthetase. In contrast Imiquimod is an imidazoquinonin tetracyclicamine which alters the immune response by possibly inducing interferon alpha.

Q4. Answer D

Glansectomy with a split-thickness skin graft would be the standard operation in the UK. Penile preserving surgery has proven equivalent oncological outcomes to radical surgery with the benefits of improved sexual, urinary and psychological results. Radical radiotherapy tends to be reserved for older patients not fit for surgery or for patients who have refused surgery. This is mainly due to its higher recurrence rate (up to 40%) and associated morbidity, which includes penile necrosis requiring amputation.

Q5. Answer C

In patients with clinically impalpable inguinal nodes at presentation, around 20% will harbour occult lymph node metastases. If all patients went onto have inguinal lymph node dissections 80% would be over treated and exposed to the morbidity of surgery. In an attempt to identify the 20% of patients with metastatic disease and avoid the unnecessary morbidity in the other 80% the technique of DSLNB was developed.

It is well accepted that penile cancers spread by embolisation via the lymphatics in a predictable stepwise fashion to the inguinal and then to the iliac nodes. The concept of sentinel lymph node biopsy was first described in men with penile cancer in 1977 by Cabanas. Unfortunately, due to a high false negative rate (FNR) and lack of reproducibility the technique fell out of favour until several modifications were made in the mid 1990s. The FNR of the DSLNB technique in penile cancer patients has been reduced to around 5%. The technique has been shown to be reproducible and has a short learning curve in the hands of penile cancer centres.

To identify the SLN pre operative mapping with Technetium 99m (Tc99m) labelled nanocolloid is essential. Intra operatively a handheld gamma probe is used to detect the 'hot' nodes and injected patent blue dye helps visualise the SLNs. The addition of preoperative ultrasound and fine needle aspiration cytology, intraoperative palpation and immunohistochemical stains have also helped to reduce the FNR.

Q6. Answer B

Medial border of adductor longus muscle is not an anatomical boundary it's the lateral border. The inguinal ligament superiorly, the medial border of sartorius muscle laterally, the lateral border of adductor longus muscle and tendon medially. The floor comprises the iliopsoas muscle laterally, the pectineus muscle medially and the femoral vessels.

Q7. Answer E

Tumour location does not influence risk of metastatic disease, all the others do. The most important risk factors appear to be sarcomatoid and basaloid variants, higher grade, perineural and vascular invasion.

Q8. Answer C

It is known that the majority of local, regional and distant recurrence occurs in the first 2 years following initial treatment. Follow up is therefore intense for this period and then relaxed to every 6 months out to 5 years when the majority of patients can be discharged. It's vital that patients are taught self-examination from the outset.

Q9. Answer D

All of the answers except radiotherapy are genuine treatment options in contemporary urological practice. Small areas of disease can be managed by either WLE or topical therapy with 5 FU or Imiquimod creams. Laser therapy with CO_2 or Nd:YAG has been well reported. Total glans resurfacing surgery tends to be reserved for disease refractory to the above or extensive PeIN on the glans penis. Circumcision is strongly recommended in these patients as it removes a potential site of recurrence, makes surveillance and topical treatment easier.

Q10. Answer A

Adjuvant chemotherapy is recommended for patients with good performance status and either pN2, pN3, M1 disease. Three cycles of cisplatin and fluorouracil are recommended as per 2013 EAU guidelines. Several other regimes have been tried in small series including taxanes and carboplatin.

Q11. Answer E

Prophylactic HSV vaccination. All would be potentially useful except vaccination against HSV, which has no proven causal link to penile cancer.

Q12. Answer B

HPV type 16 appears most prevalent in Europe, North and South America and India. Many studies to date have found HPV type 16 present in up to 50% of cases, when penile SCC histology has been retrospectively reviewed.

Although several risk factors for the development of penile SCC are well known (see list below) the exact pathogenesis is largely unknown. There appears to be at least two pathways, an HPV associated and a (non-HPV associated) chronic inflammatory associated pathway. The likely HPV related proteins involved are E6 and E7. They are known to bind to and inactivate the host cell tumour suppressor genes p53 and pRb both are negative regulators of cellular proliferation.

Recent work by Calmon and associates found a link between the HPV 16 related E6 protein and the ANXA1 gene. ANXA1 is one of the Annexin super family proteins involved with differentiation, apoptosis, proliferation and inflammation. It is proposed that E6 can interfere with the regulation of expression of genes by interacting and binding to TNF alpha-receptor 1, FAS-associated protein with death domain (FADD) and Caspase 8 and via degradation of pro-apoptotic BAX and BAK. Other recognised risk factors include smoking, increasing age >60 years, poor personal hygiene, phimosis (present in 25% of penile cancer patients), PUVA therapy, BXO or lichen sclerosus et atrophicus. The exact pathologic role of chronic inflammatory conditions like BXO in the aetiology of penile cancer remains largely unknown.

Q13. Answer E

Condyloma acuminatum is a predominantly a sexually transmitted infection caused by human papillomavirus (HPV) and spread through oral, anal and genital sexual contact and is therefore a benign condition. All of the other genital dermatoses are associated with penile SCC. Lichen sclerosus and Bowenoid papulosis are sporadically associated with penile SCC, whereas, Paget's disease and Buschke–Löwenstein are precancerous lesions and up to 30% transform into invasive SCC.

Q14. Answer C

PeIN affecting the glans penis or inner prepuce is referred to as erythroplasia of Queyrat (EQ). In comparison to Bowen disease it is when the skin of the penile shaft, rest of the genitalia or the perineum are affected. Management and treatment involve histopathological diagnosis and treatment options focus on penile-sparing procedures, including topical chemotherapy agents, WLE, glans resurfacing, laser therapy (CO_2, neodymium:yttrium-aluminum-garnet [Nd:YAG], potassium titanyl phosphate [KTP]) and Moh's micrographic surgery (not common practice in the UK). When the lesions are located solely on the foreskin, circumcision is often adequate for local control.

EMQs – ANSWERS

Q15. Answer B

Q16. Answer E

Q17. Answer D

Q18. Answer F

Q19. Answer A

Q20. Answer D

Penile lesions suspicious for cancer should be biopsied. Histological confirmation even in clinically obvious cases, must be obtained before definitive surgical management of the primary lesion.

In ≥G2pT1 penile SCC and impalpable inguinal nodes (cN0) staging with USS+/– FNAC followed by DSLNB is the standard of care in the UK if both USS and FNAC are negative.

Magnetic resonance imaging (MRI) with an alprostadil-induced erection is a useful imaging test to exclude corporal invasion. However, this can be unpleasant for the patient. The sensitivity and specificity of MRI in predicting corporal or urethral invasion have been reported as 82.1% and 73.6%, respectively.

Q21. Answer C

Q22. Answer A

Q23. Answer G

Q24. Answer E

The treatment choice for the primary lesion depends on tumour location, size, histology, stage, grade and patient preference. Tumours confined to the prepuce are often managed by radical circumcision only for treatment of the primary lesion.

Unfit patients with locally advanced disease (cT3/T4) are best served by radical surgery and perineal urethrostomy for treatment of the local disease.

Topical chemotherapy with 5-FU or Imiquimod is an effective first-line management for treating small (<2 cm) glanular PeIN (i.e., erythroplasia of Queyrat). Circumcision is strongly recommended prior to use of topical chemotherapy agents. Treatment surveillance must be assessed by biopsy and patients should be kept under long-term follow-up. Total or partial glans resurfacing with extragenital split-thickness skin graft reconstruction is a secondary option when topical agents have failed. Glans resurfacing may also be performed as a primary treatment modality for PeIN. The procedure involves denuding the glans penis of the epithelium and reconstructing the glans with a split-thickness skin graft. One study reported up to 20% invasive disease was found on histopathological analysis of glans resurfacing specimens for presumed PeIN.

Q25. Answer A

Q26. Answer E

Q27. Answer G

SCC accounts for 95% of penile cancers. It can be subdivided into usual type (60%–70%), papillary (7%), condylomatous (7%), basaloid (4%–10%), verrucous (7%) or sarcomatoid (1%–4%). Both sarcomatoid and basaloid subtypes are more aggressive and have a poorer prognosis. Rare tumours are malignant melanoma (2%), basal cell carcinoma (2%), sarcomas (1%) and extramammary Paget's disease (essentially adenocarcinoma arising in the penile skin apocrine glands) (1%).

Q28. Answer A

Q29. Answer B

Q30. Answer F

The incidence of penile cancer in the UK and Europe ranges from 0.1 to 0.9/100,000 men per year. This equates to around 1% of male malignancies. In Uganda and Paraguay, the incidence rises to 4.4 and 4.2/100,000 men per year, where it accounts for up to 10% of malignancy in men.

There are approximately 400 new cases of penile cancer in the UK per year. This led to the development of 10 supra-regional units managing the disease as per improving outcomes in urological cancers written by NICE in 2002, commissioned by the Department of Health. The aim is for each unit to serve a population of at least 4 million people and treat 25 new cases per year. This model not only allows greater expertise to be developed and improves patient care but also increases research collaborations to be improved.

CHAPTER 11: ANDROLOGY

Rozh Jalil and Jas S. Kalsi

MCQs

Q1. Phosphodiesterase 5 inhibitors cause:
A. Increased (nitric oxide) NO breakdown
B. Increased NO levels in penile endothelium
C. Increased disintegration of free oxygen radicals.
D. Increase cGMP levels
E. Decreases cAMP levels

Q2. Regarding Balanitis xerotica obliterans (lichen sclerosus et atrophicus):
A. Extra genital involvement never occurs.
B. Has possible auto-immune pathogenesis.
C. 50% cases of penile cancer have BXO changes.
D. It only effects older population.
E. Is an autoimmune disorder.

Q3. Regarding alprostadil pharmacotherapy in ED:
A. Prostaglandin E1 cause vasoconstriction of penile veins.
B. Intracavernosal alprostadil injection is associated with penile pain in 40% cases.
C. When priapism occurs conservative route is feasible for it resolves spontaneously in 50% cases.
D. Alprostadil increases introcavernosal nitrous oxide concentration.
E. Causes rise in cGMP levels.

Q4. Which of the following is NOT a risk of intracavernosal injection of vasoactive agents?
A. Pain
B. Fibrosis
C. Priapism
D. Urinary retention
E. Haematoma

Q5. Which answer is CORRECT regarding ED and diabetes mellitus?
A. The incidence of ED is 30%–50%.
B. The cause of ED is almost entirely vasculogenic.
C. Failure to ejaculate is common in diabetics.
D. Spontaneous nocturnal erections are preserved in most diabetics with ED.
E. Somatic sensory neuropathy is the common cause of ED.

Q6. Which of these is CORRECT regarding the effects of sildenafil?
A. Is excreted unmetabolised in urine.
B. Erythromycin increases plasma levels of sildenafil.
C. Priapism is a common side effect.
D. Discontinuation due to adverse events is higher than placebo.
E. Has a half life of eighteen hours.

Q7. All the following are TRUE for a three-piece inflatable penile prosthesis except:
A. Infection rate with penile implant is 1%–3%
B. Patients should be warned of migration, erosion and mechanical failure.
C. Penile prosthesis satisfaction rates are 70%–87%.
D. Both the flaccid penis and erection produced with prosthesis are no different than normal.
E. Infection and erosion are significantly higher in spinal cord injury patients.

Q8. The following are TRUE about Klinefelter's syndrome except:
A. Affected male has 47, XXY genotype.
B. It affects 1 in 650 males.

C. Androgen replacement may be needed as patient ages.

D. Seminomatous germ cell tumours are more common in these patients.

E. Karyotyping is used for diagnosis.

Q9. **The following are TRUE for Y microdeletions and infertility except:**

A. Y deletions are not found in normospermic man.

B. Most frequently detected microdeletion is AZFc.

C. AZFa microdeletion may cause variable phenotype ranging from azoospermia to oligozoospermia.

D. Deletions are extremely rare with sperm concentration >5 million sperms/mL.

E. Y-deletion spermatozoa will transmit the deletion to male offspring via in vitro fertilisation (IVF) or intracytoplasmic sperm injection (ICSI)

Q10. **Peyronie's disease**

A. Is more common in the Afro-Caribbean population.

B. Is associated with diabetes.

C. Complex surgical correction always performed with saphenous vein grafts.

D. Is associated with TGF-α.

E. Salvage surgery has poor results.

EMQs

Q11–16. **Semen analysis**

A. <4% normal forms

B. <32% motile sperms

C. <15 million/mL

D. 39

E. ≥7.2

F. 15

G. >1.5

For each of the following descriptions, select the most appropriate diagnosis. Each option may be used once, more than once or not at all.

Q11. **Oligozoospermia**

Q12. **Asthenozoospermia**

Q13. **Teratozoospermia**

Q14. **Lower limit of normal semen volume (mL)**

Q15. **Lower limit of normal for sperm concentration (10^6 per mL)**

Q16. **Semen pH**

Q17–20. **Spermatogenic failure**

A. Raised FSH, LH and low testosterone

B. Raised FSH

C. Normal FSH level

D. Likelihood of sperm retrieval is zero

E. No effect on spermatogenesis

For each of the following descriptions, select the most appropriate diagnosis. Each option may be used once, more than once or not at all.

Q17. **Testicular deficiency**

Q18. **Absent spermatogonia**

Q19. **Normal numbers of spermatogonia**

Q20. **AZFa and AZFb microdeletions**

Q21–26. **Genetic disorders in infertility**

A. Female external genitalia and absence of pubic hair

B. Partial androgen insensitivity syndrome

C. Predominant form is X-linked recessive disorder

D. 47, XXY

E. </=10 millions spermatozoa/mL

F. 5.8%

G. 10%

For each of the following descriptions, select the most appropriate diagnosis. Each option may be used once, more than once or not at all.

Q21. Incidence of chromosomal abnormalities in infertile men

Q22. Higher incidence of autosomal abnormalities (10 times)

Q23. Klinefelter's syndrome

Q24. Kallman syndrome

Q25. Reifenstein syndrome

Q26. Complete androgen insensitivity syndrome (CAIS)

Q27–31. Cystic fibrosis (CF) and male infertility
   A. 2%
   B. Autosomal-recessive disorder
   C. Chest infections
   D. CFTR
   E. Chromosome 3
   F. Chromosome 7
   G. Autosomal dominant disorder
   H. 10%

For each of the following descriptions, select the most appropriate answer. Each option may be used once, more than once or not at all.

Q27. Mode of inheritance of cystic fibrosis

Q28. The percentage of patients with obstructive azoospermia and congenital bilateral absence of the vas deferens (CBAVD) in association with CFTR mutations.

Q29. Common symptom in patients with cystic fibrosis

Q30. Test in patients with CBAVD

Q31. The location of CF transmembrane conductance regulator (CFTR) gene

Q32–37. Azoospermia
   A. 15%–20%
   B. Normal testicular volume and FSH levels
   C. 15%
   D. 1%–3%
   E. Absent fructose with acidic semen
   F. Absent mannose with alkaline semen
   G. 50%

For each of the following descriptions, select the most appropriate answer. Each option may be used once, more than once or not at all.

Q32. Percentage of patients with azoospermia having obstructive azoospermia.

Q33. Men with obstructive azoospermia.

Q34. Percentage of patients with azoospermia having intratesticular obstruction.

Q35. Percentage of patients with obstructive azoospermia having ejaculatory duct obstruction.

Q36. Ejaculatory duct obstruction

Q37. Successful sperm retrieval in Sertoli cell only syndrome using micro-dissection TESE

Q38–43. Vasectomy
   A. 9.2%
   B. 97%
   C. 88%
   D. 17%
   E. Up to 5%
   F. 0.51%
   G. 0.28%

For each of the following descriptions, select the most appropriate diagnosis. Each option may be used once, more than once or not at all.

Q38. People regretting their decision to have vasectomy

Q39. Microsurgical vasectomy reversal patency rates for an interval up to 3 years

Q40. Microsurgical vasectomy reversal patency rates for an interval of 3–8 years

Q41. Acute local complications associated with vasectomy

Q42. Early recanalisation after ligation

Q43. Early recanalisation after cauterisation

Q44–51. Drugs for erectile dysfunction
   A. Tadalafil
   B. Vardenafil
   C. Apomorphine

D. Pentoxifylline
E. Testosterone
F. Alprostadil
G. Alpha-blockers
H. Sildenafil
I. Beta blockers

For each of the following descriptions, select the most appropriate diagnosis. Each option may be used once, more than once or not at all.

Q44. Exhibits inhibition of both PDE5 and PDE11.

Q45. Has half life of 4 hours.

Q46. Works by acting on central dopaminergic receptors.

Q47. Is a non-specific phosphodiesterase inhibitor.

Q48. Is contraindicated in men with sleep apnoea syndrome.

Q49. Comes in intraurethral and intramuscular forms.

Q50. Sildenafil should not be taken within four hours following treatment with?

Q51. Patients with hereditary degenerative retinal disorders are contra-indicated to?

Q52–56. Varicocele
A. Does increase the chance of sponta-neous pregnancy
B. Does not increase the chance of spontaneous pregnancy
C. Microsurgical technique
D. 5%
E. Visible on standing
F. 11%
G. Embolisation
H. Palpable on standing

For each of the following descriptions, select the most appropriate answer. Each option may be used once, more than once or not at all.

Q52. Percentage of adults affected by varicocele

Q53. Least recurrence rates recorded after

Q54. Incidence of hydrocele after high ligation

Q55. Grade 3 varicocele

Q56. Repair of subclinical varicocele

Q57–62. Erectile dysfunction
A. 3% infection rate
B. Aphrodisiac
C. Yawning
D. Half life 2.6–3.7 hours
E. Back ache and myalgia
F. 41% drop-out rate

For each of the following descriptions, select the most appropriate answer. Each option may be used once, more than once or not at all.

Q57. Tadalafil

Q58. Sildenafil

Q59. Apomorphine

Q60. Yohimbine

Q61. Penile prosthesis

Q62. Alprostadil

Q63–67. Erectile dysfunction
A. Erectile dysfunction
B. Premature ejaculation
C. Phosphodiesterase 11
D. Nerve-sparing radical prostatectomy
E. Phosphodiesterase 5 inhibitors are metabolised
F. Cyclo-oxygenase pathway

For each of the following descriptions, select the most appropriate answer. Each option may be used once, more than once or not at all.

Q63. Incidence increases with ageing.

Q64. Incidence remains the same irrespective of age.

Q65. Skeletal muscles.

Q66. Preservation of cavernosal nerves from the autonomic pelvic plexus.

Q67. Cytochrome P450.

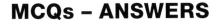

MCQs – ANSWERS

Q1. Answer D

NO is released either at non-adrenergic non-cholinergic nerve terminals (nitrergic) on the cavernous smooth muscle cell or on the endothelial cell lining of the sinusoids. Through membrane-bound G proteins, NO activates guanylate cyclase, which induces cleavage of guanosine triphosphate to 3′,5′-cyclic guanosine monophosphate (3′,5′-cGMP). The smooth muscle-relaxing effects of NO are mediated by this second messenger (cGMP). Cyclic GMP activates protein kinase G, which phosphorylates proteins at the so-called maxi-potassium channels. This results in an outflow of potassium ions into the extracellular space with subsequent hyperpolarisation, with inhibition of voltage-dependent calcium channels and therefore a decrease in intracellular calcium ion concentrations. The intracellular decline in calcium ions suppresses the activity of myosin light chain kinase and thus increases the intracellular content of dephosphorylated myosin light chain, which enables the smooth muscle cell to relax. The enzyme phosphodiesterase type 5 inactivates cGMP and thereby reduces relaxation. By inhibiting this enzyme, PDE5 inhibitors promote smooth muscle relaxation in the corpus cavernosum by increasing the cGMP concentration.

Q2. Answer B

Extra genital disease can occur, though in contrast to women, perianal disease is uncommon in men; 28% patients with penile carcinoma have histological changes of lichen sclerosis [1]. The condition occurs in all ages.

Q3. Answer B

Prostaglandin E1 causes direct relaxation of cavernosal smooth muscle and antagonises the action of norepinephrine. These dual effects may explain its efficacy in inducing erections. The Alprostadil Study Group reported a 2% incidence of penile fibrosis. Pain is the major problem associated with alprostadil injection, with an incidence of 16% to 40% and a clear dose dependency. Alprostadil has a higher rate of penile pain compared to papaverine. Prolonged erection occurred in 5% of the men in the Alprostadil Study Group [2].

Q4. Answer D

Intracavernosal injection of vasoactive agents carries the risk of fibrosis, penile pain, prolonged erection, priapism and hematoma at the injection site. Fibrosis of the corpus cavernosum is a particular concern with papaverine [2].

Q5. Answer A

In diabetics, the incidence of ED is estimated to range from 35% to 50%. The cause of ED in diabetes mellitus is multifactorial. Anejaculation and retrograde ejaculation can occur in diabetic patients due to autonomic neuropathy [3].

Q6. Answer B

Sildenafil is extensively metabolised by cytochrome P450 3A4 and 2C9. Drugs that inhibit these isoenzymes may increase sildenafil plasma levels. Erythromycin, a CYP3A4 inhibitor, has been shown to increase plasma sildenafil concentrations by 182%. Sildenafil has a low incidence of adverse effects, and these side effects are generally transient and mild to moderate in nature. In clinical trials the most common side effects were headache (16%), flushing (10%) and dyspepsia (7%). Some patients (about 3%) also reported changes in vision, predominantly colour tinge to vision, but also increased sensitivity to light or blurred vision. No cases of priapism were reported. The discontinuation rate due to adverse events among the treated patients was not significantly different from those receiving placebo (2.5% vs. 2.3%).

Q7. Answer D

The infection rates for penile prosthesis are 1%–3%. The patient considering prosthesis implantation should be informed of the possibilities of infection and erosion, mechanical failure and migration of the device that usually require reoperation. Both the appearance of the flaccid penis and the erection produced by prostheses are different than normal. Penile prosthesis satisfaction rates are high (70%–87%) [4].

Q8. Answer D

The Klinefelter's syndrome is the most frequent sex chromosome abnormality. Testosterone levels may be normal or low. Germ cell presence and sperm production are variable in men with Klinefelter's mosaicism, 46,XY/47,XXY. These patients have 50 times higher risk of germ cell tumours which usually contains non-seminomatous germ cells and present at an earlier age and seldom are gonadal in location.

Q9. Answer C

Y deletions (Yq11 micro-deletions) were not found in normospermic men and thus have a clear-cut cause effect relationship with spermatogenic failure. The highest frequency is found in azoospermic men (8%–12%) followed by oligospermic (3%–7%) men. Deletions are extremely rare with a sperm concentration >5 millions of spermatozoa/mL. (approximately 0.7%).
The most frequently deleted region is AZFc (approximately 65%–70%), followed by deletions of the AZFb and AZFb+c or AZFa+b+c regions (25%–30%) whereas deletions of the AZFa region are extremely rare (5%). The complete removal of the AZFa and AZFb regions is associated with severe testicular phenotype, Sertoli cell-only syndrome and spermatogenic arrest, respectively. The complete removal of the AZFc region causes a variable phenotype which may range from azoospermia to oligozoospermia. Classical AZF deletions do not confer risk for cryptorchidism or testis cancer.

Q10. Answer B

Peyronie's disease is a connective tissue disorder involving the growth of fibrous plaques in tunica albuginea of the penis. It affects up to 10% of all men. It's more common in Caucasian men over the age of 40. It is associated with diabetes mellitus and smoking. There is evidence to suggest that the inflammation associated with Peyronie's is at least partly mediated through the action of TGFβ. Pentoxifylline a possible medical treatment option is a TGβ1 inhibitor.

Surgery is very effective at correcting the curvature when the disease is in the chronic phase (93% success using plaque incision and grafting). Penile shortening greater than 1 cm occurred in only 25% and new onset ED in 15% [5]. Even when previous surgery has failed salvage surgery in expert hand has a high success rate [6]. A number of different graft materials have been used with success [7].

EMQs – ANSWERS

Q11. Answer C

Q12. Answer B

Q13. Answer A

Q14. Answer G

Q15. Answer F

Q16. Answer E

Semen analysis specimens should be collected over the period of few weeks after 2–5 days of sexual abstinence. The specimen should be delivered within 1 hour to the laboratory. The WHO has standardised the normal values for semen parameters as shown in the following table.

Parameter	Lower reference limit (range)
Semen volume (mL)	1.5 (1.4–1.7)
Total sperm number (10^6 per ejaculate)	39 (33–46)
Sperm concentration (10^6 per mL)	15 (12–16)
Total motility (PR + NP)	40 (38–42)
Progressive motility (PR, %)	32 (31–34)
Vitality (live spermatozoa, %)	58 (55–63)
Sperm morphology (normal forms, %)	4 (3.0–4.0)
Other consensus threshold values	
pH > 7.2	
Peroxidase-positive leukocytes (106 per mL)	<1.0
MAR test (motile spermatozoa with bound particles, %)	<50
Immunobead test (motile spermatozoa with bound beads, %)	<50
Seminal zinc (μmol/ejaculate)	>2.4
Seminal fructose (μmol/ejaculate)	>13
Seminal neutral glucosidase (mU/ejaculate)	>20

Q17. Answer A

Q18. Answer B

Q19. Answer C

Q20. Answer D

Testicular deficiency of spermatogenic failure can present as non-obstructive azoospermia or oligo-astheno-teratozoospermia. In these men hypergonadotropic hypogonadism is present denoted by raised FSH, LH and sometimes low testosterone levels. FSH is usually elevated in the absence of Spermatogonia. In maturation arrest where the spermatogonia are normal then FSH levels are usually normal. Microdeletions on the long arm of the Y chromosomes (Yq11) can be associated with infertility. Y deletions are not seen in normospermic men. AZFc is most common followed by AZFb and AZFa being least common. Complete removal of AZFa and AZFb is associated with Sertoli only syndrome while AZFc deletion can present as oligozoospermia to azoospermia.

Q21. Answer F

Q22. Answer E

Q23. Answer D

Q24. Answer C

Q25. Answer B

Q26. Answer A

Klinefelter's syndrome (47,XXY) is the most frequent sex chromosome abnormality. Testosterone levels are normal or low. Androgen replacement may be needed in these men as they age. Germ cell presence and sperm production are variable in patients with mosaicism (46,XY/47,XXY). All patients of Klinefelter's syndrome who have undergone sperm retrieval should have a long-term endocrinological review. Kallman syndrome is the most common X-linked disorder in infertility. It is X-linked recessive disorder (mutation in KALIG1 gene on Xp22.3). these patients have hypogonadotropic hypogonadism with anosmia and infertility. Spermatogenesis can be induced by hormonal treatment. Reifenstein syndrome is a state of partial androgen insensitivity with predominantly male phenotype including micropenis, perineal hypospadias and cryptorchidism. Complete androgen insensitivity syndrome (Morris syndrome), the phenotype is of female external genitalia and absence of pubic hair.

Q27. Answer B

Q28. Answer A

Q29. Answer C

Q30. Answer D

Q31. Answer F

Cystic fibrosis is an autosomal recessive disorder involving mutation of the cystic fibrosis transmembrane conductance regulator (CFTR) gene located on the short arm of chromosome 7. In Edinburgh, the percentage of patients with obstructive azoospermia and the congenital bilateral absence of the vas deferens (CBAVD) in association with CFTR mutations was 2%. CBAVD should be carefully looked for in patients with semen volume <1.5 mL and pH less than 7.0.

Q32. Answer A

Q33. Answer B

Q34. Answer C

Q35. Answer D

Q36. Answer E

Q37. Answer G

Recent studies in the USA and Europe have shown that using the newer micro-dissection TESE technique results in up to a 50% successful sperm retrieval even in patients with Sertoli cell only syndrome (SCOS). This high success in also seen in patients with previous failed retrievals elsewhere using either TESA or conventional TESE [8].

Q38. Answer A

Q39. Answer B

Q40. Answer C

Q41. Answer E

Q42. Answer F

Q43. Answer G

In a survey of vasectomised in Australia, a proportion of 9.2% of men expressed regret in regard to having had the vasectomy [9].

Rates of patency and pregnancy varies depending on the interval from the vasectomy to the reversal. If the interval had been less than 3 years, the patency was found to be 97% and pregnancy 76%, 3 to 8 years 88% and 53%, 9 to 14 years 79% and 44% and 15 years or more 71% and 30% [10].

Philp et al. [11] reviewed over 16000 vasectomy patients and found that early recanalisation was 0.51% if the vasectomy ends were ligated and 0.28% if cauterised.

Q44. Answer A

Q45. Answer B

Q46. Answer C

Q47. Answer D

Q48. Answer E

Q49. Answer F

Q50. Answer G

Q51. Answer H

Tadalafil inhibits phosphodiesterase 5 and phosphodiesterase 11 thus causing myalgia and backache. Pentoxifylline is a non-specific phosphodiesterase inhibitor used in patients with peripheral vascular disease and venous leg ulcers. It has also been used in treating Peyronie's disease (unlicensed) [12].

Q52. Answer F

Q53. Answer C

Q54. Answer D

Q55. Answer E

Q56. Answer B

Varicocele is present in 11% of adult males and in 25% of men with abnormal semen analysis. Meta-analysis by Agarwal et al. showed that surgical treatment of clinical varicocele significantly improved semen parameters [13]. The Ever's meta-analysis concluded that there is no evidence that the varicocele treatment improves the conception rate [14]. The recurrence rate after microsurgical technique is 0.8%–4% [15].

Q57. Answer E

Q58. Answer D

Q59. Answer C

Q60. Answer B

Q61. Answer A

Q62. Answer F

Penile prosthesis implantation has one of the highest satisfaction rates (70%–87%). Mechanical failure rate is less than 5% at 5 years. Infection and erosion rates are significantly higher in patients with spinal cord injury [4,12]. Yohimbine is a sympatholytic. Apomorphine is a centrally acting dopaminergic agonist and it induces yawning. Myalgia and backache are known side effects of tadalafil (5.7% and 6.5%, respectively).

Q63. Answer A

Q64. Answer B

Q65. Answer C

Q66. Answer D

Q67. Answer E

About 39% of men at the age of 40 years have erectile dysfunction rising to 67% at the age of 70 years (Massachusetts Male Ageing Study). According to National Health and Social Life Survey (NHSLS), premature ejaculation is not affected by age. Sildenafil, tadalafil and vadenafil are metabolised by Cytochrome P450 enzyme 3A4.

REFERENCES

1. Pietrzak P, Hadway P, Corbishley CM, Watkin NA. Is the association between balanitis xerotica obliterans and penile carcinoma underestimated? *BJU Int* 2006 Jul; 98(1): 74–6.
2. Linet OI, Ogrinc FG. Efficacy and safety of intracavernosal alprostadil in men with erectile dysfunction. The Alprostadil Study Group. *N Engl J Med* 1996 Apr 4; 334(14): 873–7.
3. Kalsi JS, Ralph DJ, Madge DJ, Kell PD, Cellek S. A comparative study of sildenafil, NCX-911 and BAY41-2272 on the anococcygeus muscle of diabetic rats. *Int J Impot Res* 2004 Dec; 16(6): 479–85.
4. Carson CC, III, Mulcahy JJ, Harsch MR. Long-term infection outcomes after original antibiotic impregnated inflatable penile prosthesis implants: Up to 7.7 years of followup. *J Urol* 2011 Feb; 185(2): 614–8.
5. Kalsi J, Minhas S, Christopher N, Ralph D. The results of plaque incision and venous grafting (Lue procedure) to correct the penile deformity of Peyronie's disease. *BJU Int* 2005 May; 95(7): 1029–33.
6. Muneer A, Kalsi J, Christopher N, Minhas S, Ralph DJ. Plaque incision and grafting as a salvage after a failed Nesbit procedure for Peyronie's disease. *BJU Int* 2004 Oct; 94(6): 878–80.
7. Kalsi JS, Christopher N, Ralph DJ, Minhas S. Plaque incision and fascia lata grafting in the surgical management of Peyronie's disease. *BJU Int* 2006 Jul; 98(1): 110–4.
8. Kalsi J, Thum MY, Muneer A, Abdullah H, Minhas S. In the era of micro-dissection sperm retrieval (m-TESE) is an isolated testicular biopsy necessary in the management of men with non-obstructive azoospermia? *BJU Int* 2012 Feb; 109(3): 418–24.
9. Holden CA, McLachlan RI, Cumming R, Wittert G, Handelsman DJ, de Kretser DM, Pitts M. Sexual activity, fertility and contraceptive use in middle-aged and older men: Men in Australia, Telephone Survey (MATeS). *Hum Reprod* 2005 Dec; 20(12): 3429–34.
10. Belker AM, Thomas AJ, Fuchs EF, Konnak JW, Sharlip ID. Results of 1,469 microsurgical vasectomy reversals by the vasovasostomy study group. *J Urol* 1991, 145(3): 505–11.

11. Philp T, Guillebaud I, Budd D. Complications of vasectomy: review of 16000 patients. *Br J Urol*, 1984; 56: 745–8.

12. Kalsi JS, Kell PD. Update on oral treatments for male erectile dysfunction. *J Eur Acad Dermatol Venereol* 2004 May; 18(3): 267–74.

13. Agarwal A, Deepinder F, Cocuzza M, Agarwal R, Short RA, Sabanegh E, et al. Efficacy of varicocelectomy in improving semen parameters: new meta-analytical approach. *Urology* 2007 Sep; 70(3): 532–8.

14. Evers JH, Collins J, Clarke J. Surgery or embolisation for varicoceles in subfertile men. *Cochrane Database Syst Rev* 2009; (1): CD000479.

15. Goldstein M, Gilbert BR, Dicker AP, Dwosh J, Gnecco C. Microsurgical inguinal varicocelectomy with delivery of the testis: an artery and lymphatic sparing technique. *J Urol* 1992 Dec; 148(6): 1808–11.

CHAPTER 12: BENIGN PROSTATIC HYPERPLASIA (BPH) AND LOWER URINARY TRACT SYMPTOMS (LUTS)

Hamid Abboudi, Jas S. Kalsi and Tev Aho

MCQs

Q1. What percentage of total serum testosterone is unbound in plasma?
A. 2%
B. 12%
C. 32%
D. 42%
E. 8%

Q2. Which of the following is TRUE with respect to BPH?
A. Is a histological process predominantly characterised by benign prostatic hypertrophy.
B. Always causes lower urinary tract symptoms.
C. May not produce bladder outlet obstruction.
D. Requires the absence of androgens.
E. Is always a progressive disease.

Q3. The following are true regarding the zonal anatomy of the prostate, EXCEPT:
A. There are four zones (central, transition zone, peripheral zone, anterior fibromuscular septum).
B. BPH mainly affects the peripheral zone.
C. The peripheral zone comprises 65% of glandular tissue of the prostate.
D. The transition comprises around 10% of the glandular tissue.
E. The majority of cancers are located in the peripheral zone.

Q4. Which of the following is FALSE regarding the International Prostate Symptom Score?
A. The questionnaire has eight questions.
B. The first seven questions are graded from 1 to 5.

C. Includes a question grading the symptom of intermittent flow.
D. A score of 8 signifies moderate LUTS.
E. A score of 20 signifies severe LUTS.

Q5. The following therapies for BPH are NOT recommended by NICE (CG97).
A. Alpha-blockers in combination with 5 alpha reductase inhibitors
B. Millin's prostatectomy
C. Bipolar TURP
D. Transurethral vaporisation of the prostate
E. Holmium laser ablation of the prostate

Q6. The following investigations are not routinely recommended for the specialist assessment of bothersome LUTS by NICE (CG97).
A. Flow rate
B. Post-void residual
C. Symptom score
D. Frequency volume chart
E. Ultrasound of renal tract

Q7. With reference to the MTOPS trial, which of the following is TRUE?
A. Single centre randomised double blinded controlled trial
B. Had the following four arms: placebo, tamsulosin, finasteride and combination
C. Defined an IPSS score increase in 4 or more as a secondary outcome
D. Defined stress incontinence as a primary outcome
E. Revealed a relative risk reduction in acute urinary retention of 81% in the combination arm compared with placebo

Q8. With reference to the PLESS trial, which of the following is NOT TRUE?
   A. Inclusion criteria included moderate-to-severe LUTS
   B. 57% relative risk reduction in AUR with finasteride compared to placebo
   C. Number needed to treat to prevent 1 episode of retention was 25
   D. Incidence of high-grade malignancy was higher in the finasteride arm
   E. Acute retention developed in 3% of men on finasteride over 4 years

Q9. Which of the following are important predictors for clinical progression of BPH?
   A. Age > 75
   B. PSA > 1.3 ng/mL
   C. $Q_{max} < 12$
   D. Prostate volume > 40 g
   E. Chronic inflammation of the prostate

Q10. Anticholinergics are contraindicated in the following, EXCEPT
   A. Post-void residual > 150 mL
   B. Patients with open angle glaucoma
   C. Toxic megacolon
   D. Patients with untreated narrow-angle glaucoma
   E. Patients with surgically treated closed-angle glaucoma

Q11. An 82-year-old man with mixed storage and voiding LUTS is referred for urodynamics. His Q_{max} is 15 mL/s and a pdet at Q_{max} of 85 cm H_2O. What is the bladder outlet obstruction index for this man?
   A. 45
   B. 50
   C. 55
   D. 70
   E. 103

Q12. An 82-year-old man with daytime frequency, urinary urgency, occasional incontinence and nocturia is treated with an anticholinergic. His incontinence worsens. Urinalysis is normal. The next step is:
   A. PVR
   B. Uroflowmetry
   C. Cystoscopy
   D. Urodynamics
   E. Renal tract ultrasound

EMQs

Q11–15. Management options for LUTS/BPH
   A. Lifestyle and fluid management
   B. Saw palmetto
   C. Tamsulosin
   D. Finasteride
   E. Tamsulosin and finasteride
   F. TURP
   G. Open prostatectomy
   H. Cystolitholopaxy
   I. Intermittent self-catheterisation
   J. Indwelling catheterisation

Regarding the clinical scenarios described below, please choose the most appropriate treatment option, from the list above. Each answer may be used once, more than once or not at all.

Q11. A 68-year-old man with no significant co-morbidities and no drug history with bothersome LUTS, IPSS score of 19, Q_{max} of 9 mL/s, prostate volume of 45 cc.

Q12. A 71-year-old man with no co-morbidities has mild LUTS with a prostate volume of 60 cc.

Q13. A 56-year-old man with IPSS 17, 25 g prostate and a PSA of 1.0 ng/mL.

Q14. A 61-year-old man with recurrent episodes of retention, and who is keen to maintain sexual function and avoid side effects of pharmacological therapies.

Q15. A 74-year-old man with no significant co-morbidities is found to have a 5-cm bladder calculus and recurrent UTIs. He also has a 90 g prostate.

Q16–21. Investigations of men with LUTS
   A. PSA
   B. Uroflowmetry
   C. eGFR
   D. Urodynamics
   E. Video urodynamics
   F. Ultrasound scan of renal tract
   G. CT urogram
   H. CT abdomen and pelvis with contrast
   I. MRI pelvis

For each of the clinical scenarios described below, what is the most appropriate next investigation that should be performed, from the list above. Each answer may be used once, more than once or not at all.

Q16. A 64-year-old man with acute urinary retention has a serum creatinine of 180.

Q17. A 41-year-old man with predominantly voiding lower urinary tract symptoms, which has not improved with self-help measures.

Q18. A 31-year-old man with an IPSS of 29.

Q19. An 82-year-old man with a history of nocturnal enuresis, PSA of 190 and creatinine of 210.

Q20. A 53-year-old male with mild LUTS and visible haematuria.

Q21. A 45-year-old man with urgency, frequency, urgency incontinence and poor stream.

Q22–25. Epidemiology of benign prostatic hyperplasia
   A. 6%
   B. 30%–40%
   C. 50%
   D. 60%–70%
   E. 80%–90%
   F. >95%

For the statements listed below, what is the most accurate answer, in the list above. Each answer may be used once, more than once or not at all.

Q22. Incidence of pathological BPH in a 71- to 80-year-old male

Q23. Percentage of patients with a maximum flow rate of <10 who will have urodynamic bladder outflow obstruction

Q24. Risk of long-term incontinence following TURP

Q25. In the MTOPS study, the risk of relative risk reduction of progression of disease with combination therapy compared with placebo

MCQs – ANSWERS

Q1. Answer A

Testosterone in blood is bound to strongly to SHBG and loosely to albumin. Only 1%–4% is free. Testosterone is loosely bound to albumin (and other plasma proteins) and therefore forms part of the bioavailable testosterone (BAT). Serum hormone binding globulin (SHBG) binds to 2/3 of the total testosterone. Free testosterone measures the free fraction, bioavailable testosterone includes free plus the weakly bound to albumin. Di-hydro testosterone (DHT) is the major form of androgens found within the prostate gland, the concentration is five times that of testosterone. Testosterone is converted to DHT by the action of 5 alpha reductase.

Q2. Answer C

Benign prostatic hyperplasia is a histological process characterised by an increase in the number of epithelial and stromal cells in the periurethral area of the prostate. New gland formation is usually only seen in the foetus, which has led to the theory of 'embryonic reawakening'. The increase in cell number may be due to cellular proliferation or apoptosis or a combination of the two. The development of BPH requires androgens during prostate development, puberty and aging. Patients castrated prior to puberty do not develop BPH. Hald's 3-ring diagram originally described the relationship between hyperplasia, prostatism and obstruction. It has now been modified to include the relationship between LUTS, BPE and BOO: only 25%–50% of men with BPH have LUTS.

Q3. Answer B

There are four zones (central zone, transition zone, peripheral zone and anterior fibromuscular septum). BPH first develops in the periurethral transition zone of the prostate. Nodular hyperplasia is an early phase of the disease, and in the later phase, the size of the nodules increases with the enlargement of glandular nodules. Alpha 1a is the most abundant adrenoreceptor subtype in the prostate. The transition zone comprises 10% of the glandular tissue, whilst the peripheral zone constitutes 65%. The remaining tissue is stroma. Most cancers arise in the peripheral zone.

Q4. Answer B

The IPSS is a validated questionnaire adopted from the AUA symptom score with an additional quality of life score. There are seven questions graded 0–5 and a single quality of life question graded 0–6. LUTS can be categorised into mild (0–7), moderate (8–19) and severe (20–35).

Q5. Answer E

The NICE LUTS guidance (May 2010) recommended that if offering surgery for managing voiding LUTS presumed secondary to BPE, do not offer minimally invasive treatments (including transurethral needle ablation [TUNA], transurethral microwave thermotherapy [TUMT], high-intensity focused ultrasound [HIFU], transurethral ethanol ablation of the prostate [TEAP] and laser coagulation) as an alternative to TURP, TUVP or HoLEP (Jones et al., 2010).

Q6. Answer E

The NICE LUTS guidance 2010 recommends that in the specialist assessment of a patient with LUTS, the clinician should offer:

An assessment of general medical history to identify possible causes and co-morbidities, including a review of all current medication (including herbal and over-the-counter medication) that may be contributing to the problem

A physical examination guided by symptoms and other medical conditions, an examination of the abdomen and external genitalia, and a DRE (Jones et al., 2010).

Further tests include a flow rate and post-void residual volume measurement as well as a urinary frequency volume chart. Men should be offered information, advice and time to decide if they wish to have PSA testing if; their LUTS are suggestive of benign prostatic enlargement or the prostate gland feels abnormal or they are concerned about prostate cancer.

The guidance only recommends a cystoscopy and/or imaging of the upper urinary tract when there is a history of recurrent infection, sterile pyuria, haematuria, pain or chronic retention.

Q7. Answer E

This study was a long-term, multi-centre double-blind trial (mean follow-up, 4.5 years) involving 3047 men to compare the effects of placebo, doxazosin, finasteride and combination therapy on measures of the clinical progression of benign prostatic hyperplasia.

The risk of overall clinical progression (primary end points) – defined as an increase above base line of at least four points in the American Urological Association symptom score, acute urinary retention, urinary incontinence, renal insufficiency or recurrent urinary tract infection – was significantly reduced by doxazosin (39% reduction and finasteride (34%), as compared with placebo. The reduction in risk associated with combination therapy (66% for the comparison with placebo) was significantly greater than that associated with doxazosin or finasteride therapy alone. The risks of acute urinary retention and the need for invasive therapy were significantly reduced by combination therapy and finasteride but not by doxazosin (McConnell et al., 2003).

Q8. Answer D

This was a double-blind, randomised, placebo-controlled trial, where 3040 men with moderate-to-severe urinary symptoms and enlarged prostate glands were treated daily with 5 mg of finasteride or placebo for four years. They were assessed with symptom scores, urinary flow rates, and the occurrence of outcome events every four months. Prostate volume was measured in a subgroup of the men. During the four-year study period, 10% in the placebo group and 5% in the finasteride group underwent surgery for benign prostatic hyperplasia (reduction in risk with finasteride, 55%). Acute urinary retention developed in 7% in the placebo group and in 3% in the finasteride group (reduction in risk with finasteride, 57%). The mean decreases in the symptom score were 3.3 in the finasteride group and 1.3 in the placebo group. Treatment with finasteride also significantly improved urinary flow rates and reduced prostate volume (McConnell et al., 1998).

It was the Prostate Cancer Prevention Trial (PCPT) that reported that 7 years of administration of finasteride reduced the risk of prostate cancer by 25% but with an apparent increased risk of high disease (Thompson et al., 2003).

Q9. Answer E

A number of risk factors have been identified which can help predict disease progression in individual patients. An increased chance of disease progression is associated with age >70, symptom severity (IPSS > 7), reduced urinary flow rate (Q_{max} <10 mL/sec) and prostate size (>30 cc).

Data from placebo arms of large drug trials has shown that PSA is an independent marker of disease progression. A PSA level of 1.4 ng/dL or higher indicates an increased risk of disease progression (McConnell et al., 2003).

The Olmsted County study measured the prevalence of symptoms of BPH in men aged 40–80. An average AUA symptom score deterioration of 0.18/yr was observed across the study with the fastest rate of deterioration observed in the 60–69 age group. Age greater than 70 is associated with a significant increase in risk of progression (Jacobsen et al., 1997).

Inflammation also appears to be important in the pathogenesis and progression of BPH. The risk of urinary retention has been found to be significantly greater in men with acute and/or chronic intraprostatic inflammation (ACI) than in those without.

Q10. Answer B

Anticholinergics, such as oxybutynin chloride, are contraindicated in patients with untreated angle closure glaucoma since anticholinergic drugs may aggravate this condition. It is also contraindicated in partial or complete obstruction of the gastrointestinal tract, hiatus hernia severe gastroesophageal reflux, paralytic ileus, toxic megacolon complicating ulcerative colitis, severe colitis and myasthenia gravis. It is also contraindicated in patients with obstructive uropathy and in patients with unstable cardiovascular status in acute haemorrhage.

Q11. Answer C

When performing urodynamics the diagnosis of bladder outlet obstruction is made by plotting the maximum flow rate (Q_{max}) against detrusor pressure at Q_{max} ($pdetQ_{max}$) into the International Continence Society Nomogram. The degree of obstruction is calculated using the Bladder Outlet Obstruction Index (BOOI) equation: $BOOI = pdet@Q_{max} - 2Q_{max}$.

If the BOOI is >40 then the patient is obstructed, if it is below 20 then the patient is unlikely to be obstructed and between 20–40 the findings are equivocal.

Q12. Answer A

LUTS in the elderly may be secondary to a number of medical conditions, including immobility, congestive cardiac failure and diabetes. Antimuscarinic agents may cause or worsen urinary incontinence in elderly patients with poor detrusor contractility. This may present with new or worsened incontinence due to overflow after the initiation of an antimuscarinic agent. This can be diagnosed with the non-invasive measurement of a PVR. Renal ultrasound is not indicated. There is no need at this point to proceed to uroflowmetry, urodynamics or cystoscopy, but these may be useful in further evaluation.

EMQs – ANSWERS

Q11. Answer E

Q12. Answer A

Q13. Answer C

Q14. Answer I

Q15. Answer G

NICE guidelines recommend pharmacotherapy only to men with bothersome LUTS when conservative management options have been unsuccessful or not appropriate. Phytotherapy is currently not recommended in the management of men with LUTS due to the heterogeneity of the products available and methodological limitations of published trials and meta-analyses.

An alpha-blocker should be offered to men with moderate to severe LUTS. Whilst a 5 alpha reductase inhibitor is most effective in men at high risk of progression and who have prostates estimated to be larger than 30 cc or PSA >1.4.

Data from the MTOPS trial would favour the use of combination therapy in the context of moderate–severe LUTS and an enlarged prostate (>30cc) over monotherapy in terms of reducing overall clinical progression and risk of acute urinary retention. Alpha-blockers can cause dizziness, postural hypotension, asthenia, nasal congestion and retrograde ejaculation. Whilst 5-alpha reductase inhibitors are associated with reduced libido, erectile dysfunction, reduced ejaculate volume and rarely rash and breast symptoms.

Options for the management of recurrent urinary retention include indwelling catheterisation, intermittent self-catheterisation (ISC) or bladder outflow surgery. However only ISC will preserve sexual function. Prostatic urethral lift procedures such as Urolift™ are currently not licensed in the context of urinary retention.

In patients with large bladder stones with significant BPH an open procedure may allow treatment of both conditions. However, a staged procedure with endoscopic/laser Cystolitholopaxy and subsequent Holep or green light prostatectomy would not be unreasonable.

Q16. Answer F

Q17. Answer B

Q18. Answer B

Q19. Answer F

Q20. Answer G

Q21. Answer D

An ultrasound of the renal tract is indicated in the presence of urinary retention and an acute kidney injury to identify upper tract obstruction confirming an obstructive uropathy. Ultrasound is safer and more cost effective compared to CT and MRI respectively. Other indications of upper tract imaging include chronic retention, haematuria, recurrent infection, sterile pyuria, profound symptoms and loin pain.

Uroflowmetry provides a visual representation of the force of a patient's urinary stream. Key parameters are Q_{max} and flow pattern (normal bell-shaped, obstructed and plateau-shaped). Urine flow is measured in mL/s and is determined using either a spinning disc, load cell or capacitance flowmeter system. Uroflowmetry is the screening test of choice in men with LUTS. It is easy to perform, cost-effective and safe. However, it is prone to within-subject variability and therefore most guidelines recommend measuring at least two flow rates and using the highest as representing the patient's best effort. Uroflowmetry is not recommended by NICE in the primary care setting.

EAU recommendations for urodynamics include:

Men with previously unsuccessful (invasive) treatment for LUTS

When considering invasive treatment for patients who cannot void >150 mL, or have a PVR >300 mL or have bothersome predominantly voiding LUTS aged <50 or >80 years

In the context of visible haematuria upper tract imaging in the form of a renal tract ultrasound or a CT urogram and a flexible cystoscopy are warranted to exclude a malignant cause for the patient's symptoms.

Q22. Answer E

Q23. Answer E

Q24. Answer A

Q25. Answer D

Barry et al. 1984, published an autopsy series highlighting pathological presence of BPH in men aged 41–50 was 23%, 61–70 was 71%, and 82% of 71–80-year-olds. If the Q_{max} is below 10 mL/s, then the chance of having bladder outflow obstruction is 90%, however if the Q_{max} is between 10–15 mL/s, then the incidence falls to 71% or less.

In the National Prostatectomy Audit, the short-term incontinence rate was 3% and long-term rates were 6%. The risk of impotence was 30%. In the MTOPS study the relative risk reduction of progression was 66%, with a 12% absolute risk reduction. The relative risk reduction of AUR with combination therapy was 81% compared to placebo.

REFERENCES

Jacobsen, S. J., D. J. Jacobson, C. J. Girman, R. O. Roberts, T. Rhodes, H. A. Guess, and M. M. Lieber, 1997, Natural history of prostatism: Risk factors for acute urinary retention. *J. Urol.*, v. 158, no. 2, pp. 481–487.

Jones, C., J. Hill, and C. Chapple, 2010, Management of lower urinary tract symptoms in men: Summary of NICE guidance. *BMJ*, v. 340, pp. c2354.

McConnell, J. D. et al., 1998, The effect of finasteride on the risk of acute urinary retention and the need for surgical treatment among men with benign prostatic hyperplasia. Finasteride Long-Term Efficacy and Safety Study Group. *N. Engl. J. Med.*, v. 338, no. 9, pp. 557–563.

McConnell, J. D. et al., 2003, The long-term effect of doxazosin, finasteride, and combination therapy on the clinical progression of benign prostatic hyperplasia: *N. Engl. J. Med.*, v. 349, no. 25, pp. 2387–2398.

Mishra, V. C., D. J. Allen, C. Nicolaou, H. Sharif, C. Hudd, O. M. Karim, H. G. Motiwala, and M. E. Laniado, 2007, Does intraprostatic inflammation have a role in the pathogenesis and progression of benign prostatic hyperplasia? *BJU. Int.*, v. 100, no. 2, pp. 327–331.

Thompson, I. M. et al., 2003, The influence of finasteride on the development of prostate cancer. *N. Engl. J. Med.*, v. 349, no. 3, pp. 215–224.

CHAPTER 13: FEMALE AND FUNCTIONAL UROLOGY

Angela Cottrell and Hashim Hashim

MCQs

Q1. Which of the following is the most predominant muscarinic receptor in the bladder?
A. M1
B. M2
C. M3
D. M4
E. M5

Q2. Which of the following antimuscarinics has the least central nervous system side effects?
A. Oxybutynin
B. Trospium chloride
C. Solifenacin
D. Darifenacin
E. Tolterodine

Q3. Which of the following is not a contra-indication for antimuscarinic use?
A. Closed-angle glaucoma
B. Bladder outflow obstruction
C. Toxic mega-colon
D. Myasthenia gravis
E. Ulcerative colitis

Q4. Which of the following is the commonest side effect of duloxetine?
A. Hot flushes
B. Anorexia
C. Dry mouth
D. Constipation
E. Nausea

Q5. What filling speed is used during cystometry in neurogenic patients?
A. <10 mL/min
B. 10–30 mL/min
C. 30–50 mL/min
D. 50–100 mL/min
E. 100 mL/min

Q6. A male patient has a detrusor pressure at maximum flow rate of 70 cm H_2O, a maximum detrusor pressure of 80 cm H_2O and a maximum flow rate of 8 mL/sec. What is his bladder outflow obstruction index?
A. 54
B. 64
C. 72
D. 110
E. 120

Q7. A patient has a spinal cord injury at the level of T4. Which complication can develop?
A. Hypotension associated with nociceptive stimulus below the level of the spinal cord lesion
B. Hypertension associated with nociceptive stimulus below the level of the spinal cord lesion
C. Vasodilatation of the skin below the level of T4 associated with nociceptive stimulus below the level of the spinal cord lesion
D. Sweating below the level of T4 associated with nociceptive stimulus below the level of the spinal cord lesion
E. Profound headache associated with nociceptive stimulus above the level of the spinal cord lesion

Q8. Which of the following is an NIDDK criteria for interstitial cystitis?
A. Pain associated with the bladder or urinary frequency of 6 months duration
B. Desire to void with the bladder filled to 120 mL of water on cystoscopy

C. Pain associated with the bladder or urinary urgency associated with the presence of glomerulations on cystoscopy visible in at least three quadrants of the bladder

D. The presence of mast cells on histology of bladder mucosa

E. Pain associated with bladder filling and frequency

Q9. How does Cystistat (hyaluronic acid) work?

A. Direct inhibition of mast cells in the urothelium

B. Coating of the urothelium

C. Intravesical instillation of histamine antagonist aimed to replenish the GAG layer

D. Intravesical instillation of proteoglycan aimed to repair defects in the GAG layer

E. Oral therapy substituting defects in the GAG layer

Q10. What is the prevalence of overactive bladder syndrome?

A. 8%

B. 11%

C. 22%

D. 31%

E. 45%

EMQs

Q11–13. Continence definitions

A. The complaint of involuntary loss of urine associated with an increase in abdominal pressure.

B. The complaint of involuntary loss of urine on effort or on exertion, or on sneezing or coughing.

C. The complaint of involuntary leakage of urine accompanied by or immediately preceded by urgency.

D. The complaint by the patient that they void too often by day.

E. The observation of passing urine more than seven times during the day.

F. The complaint of a sudden compelling desire to pass urine which is difficult to defer.

G. Waking from sleep to pass urine.

H. The number of voids after retiring to bed.

I. The complaint of loss of urine during sleep.

J. The complaint of any loss of urine.

K. The involuntary loss of urine that is a social or hygienic problem.

L. The number of voids during the day before bed.

M. The number of times urine is passed during the main sleep period.

For the following clinical features listed below, what is the correct definition from the list above?

Q11. Nocturia

Q12. Urgency urinary incontinence

Q13. Stress urinary incontinence

Q14–16. Pharmacological therapy for incontinence

A. Antimuscarinic agent

B. Selective serotonin re-uptake inhibitor (SSRI)

C. Inhibitor of the release of acetylcholine

D. Beta-2 agonist

E. Beta-3 agonist

F. Synthetic anti-diuretic hormone

G. Serotonin noradrenaline re-uptake inhibitor (SNRI)

H. Vanilloid receptor blocker

For each drug listed below, which category does it belong to, based on the options above?

Q14. Mirabegron

Q15. Duloxetine

Q16. Desmopressin

Q17–19. Pelvic organ prolapse

A. Stage 0

B. Stage I

C. Stage II

D. Stage III

E. Stage VI

F. Stage V

For the clinical features described below, what degree of pelvic organ prolapse do each of the women have?

Q17. The bladder is 4 cm above the hymen

Q18. The rectal wall is 1 cm above the hymen

Q19. The cervix and bladder are at the hymen

Q20–22. Metabolic complications of bowel segment reconstruction

A. Augmentation jejuno-cystoplasty

B. MAINZ II

C. Stomach cystoplasty

D. Colonic neobladder

E. Appendiceal Mitrofanoff

For the following metabolic complications, choose from the list above, which type of bowel segment reconstruction that has been used.

Q20. Hypochloraemic metabolic alkalosis

Q21. Hyperchloraemic metabolic acidosis

Q22. Hypochloraemic metabolic acidosis

Q23–25. Validation of LUTS Quality of Life questionnaires

A. Content/face validity

B. Internal consistency

C. Stability (test-retest reliability)

D. Construct validity

E. Criterion validity

F. Responsiveness

There are several steps that need to be followed when validating a lower urinary tract symptoms quality of life questionnaire. Match the definitions to the term they correspond to.

Q23. Description of how well the questionnaire correlates with a 'gold standard' measure that already exists.

Q24. Extent to which items within the questionnaire are related to each other.

Q25. Whether the questionnaire measures the same sort of things in the same person over a period of time.

MCQs – ANSWERS

Q1. **Answer B**

Post-ganglionic parasympathetic nerves release acetylcholine which binds to muscarinic receptors leading to detrusor contraction. There are five types of muscarinic receptors described (M1-5). M1-3 receptors are found in the bladder. Two thirds of receptors are M2 and one-third are M3. Functionally the most important muscarinic receptor is the M3 receptor, which induce entry of calcium into the cell leading to detrusor contraction even though the M2 receptor is the most commonly found one.

Q2. **Answer B**

Whilst antimuscarinic agents are the mainstay of pharmacological treatment of overactive bladder syndrome, their use can be limited by side effects. Central nervous system effects are particularly important in the elderly population as the structure of the blood brain barrier may be impaired due to stroke, Alzheimer's disease or diabetes. Central nervous system side effects include headache, dizziness or tiredness. These may be determined by the ability of the antimuscarinic agent to cross the blood brain barrier, the specificity for muscarinic receptors or actions of metabolites. Antimuscarinics are described as tertiary (e.g., oxybutynin) or quaternary amines (e.g., trospium chloride). Tertiary amines are lipophilic and are more likely to cross the blood brain barrier compared with quaternary amines which are, in theory, associated with fewer central nervous system side effects. All the tertiary amines (darifenacin, tolterodine and solifenacin) may cause cognitive side effects and exacerbating the anticholinergic burden but oxybutynin seems to be the one with the most negative effect on cognitive function. All five muscarinic receptors are found in the brain. M1 and M2 receptors are associated with memory and cognition whereas M3 receptors (which are clinically significant for detrusor contraction) have a low expression in the brain. Antimuscarinics, which have receptor specificity for M3 receptors, in theory, should have a lower risk of cognitive side effects.

Further Reading

Wagg A, Verdejo C, Molander U. Review of cognitive impairment with antimuscarinic agents in elderly patients with overactive bladder. *Int J Clin Pract*, 2010 Aug; 64(9): 1279–1286.

Chancellor M, Boone T. Anticholinergics for overactive bladder therapy: Central nervous system effects. *CNS Neurosci Ther*, 2012 Feb; 18(2): 167–174.

Q3. **Answer B**

The use of anticholinergics is contraindicated in closed-angle glaucoma, toxic megacolon and ulcerative colitis. Myasthenia gravis is an autoimmune neurological disorder characterised by antibodies against the acetylcholine receptor. Whilst the British National Formulary describes significant bladder outflow obstruction and urinary retention as contraindications to antimuscarinic use, there is evidence that the use of antimuscarinics in patients with bladder outflow obstruction does not lead to significant adverse events. In a randomised, placebo-controlled trial, Abrams et al. investigated the safely of tolterodine in men with a urodynamic diagnosis of bladder outflow obstruction and overactive bladder syndrome. Whilst the increase in post-void residual urine was statistically higher in patients treated with tolterodine compared with placebo, this was not clinically meaningful; the rate of adverse events (including urinary retention) was not significantly higher in those taking antimuscarinic therapy, as long as post-void residuals are less than 200 mL.

Further Reading

Abrams P, Kaplan S, De Koning Gans HJ. Millard Safety and tolerability of tolterodine for the treatment of overactive bladder in men with bladder outlet obstruction. *J Urol*, 2006 Mar; 175(3 Pt 1): 999–1004.

Q4. Answer E

Duloxetine is a serotonin and noradrenaline reuptake inhibitor. Inhibition of serotonin and noradrenaline reuptake is thought to improve stress incontinence by increasing tone in the pudendal nerve, thereby increasing tone in the rhabdosphincter during bladder filling. A Cochrane Review in 2009 evaluated the use of serotonin and noradrenaline reuptake inhibitors in ten randomised controlled trials, showing a significant improvement in quality of life and reduction in incontinence episode frequency by 50% compared with placebo. Objective cure (as measured by pad test) however failed to demonstrate a benefit over placebo. Amongst the trials in this review, approximately one in three participants experienced adverse events. Side effects of duloxetine include hot flushes, anorexia, dry mouth and constipation but the commonest is nausea.

Further Reading

Mariappan P, Alhasso AA, Grant A, N'Dow JMO. Serotonin and noradrenaline reuptake inhibitors (SNRI) for stress urinary incontinence in adults (review). *Cochrane Database of Systematic Reviews* 2005; Issue 3. Art. No.: CD004742. doi:10.1002/14651858.CD004742.pub2.

Q5. Answer A

The filling rate during filling cystometry is important and determined by the patient undergoing urodynamic assessment (e.g., neuropathic versus non-neuropathic). Medium to fast fill during filling cystometry is described as 50–100 mL/min. In neuropathic bladders a slower fill of <20 mL/min is used. Fast filling in a neuropathic patient may lead to 'artefactual' detrusor contractions and reduced compliance.

Q6. Answer A

The bladder outlet obstruction index (BOOI) enables classification of patients' voiding into obstructed, unobstructed or equivocal once calculated numerically and is commonly plotted on the International Continence Society nomogram. This replaces the Abrams-Griffiths number and nomogram.

The BOOI is calculated using the following formula: $pdetQ_{max} - (2*Q_{max})$

- $pdetQ_{max}$ = detrusor pressure at maximum flow rate
- Q_{max} = maximum flow rate
- Obstructed if BOOI is >40
- Equivocal if BOOI is 20–40
- Unobstructed if BOOI is <20

Bladder contractility index can also be calculated from these variables to determine ranges of contractility using the following formula: $pdetQ_{max} + (5*Q_{max})$.

A bladder contractility index of <100 is weak, 100–150 is normal and >150 is strong contractility.

Q7. Answer B

Autonomic dysreflexia is a serious and potentially fatal complication of spinal cord injuries above the level of T6. In patients with a cord lesion above the level of T6 and an intact distal autonomous cord, noxious stimuli (such as urinary tract instrumentation, constipation or blocked catheter) lead to disordered sympathetic response. Vasoconstriction of vascular beds (including splanchnic circulation, skin and skeletal muscle) below the level of the lesion leads to hypertension. To counteract the hypertension, bradycardia may be seen; however due to the level of cord injury the normal physiological response by baroreceptors, including vasodilatation, is prohibited. Above the level of the cord lesion there is flushing and sweating. Systemic features include anxiety and nausea. Management includes preliminary preventative measures, identifying those at risk of autonomic dysreflexia and early recognition. Once it has been identified that this is a urological emergency, the patient should be sat up, triggering factors should be removed and hypertension treated with oral nifedipine, glyceryl trinitrate (GTN) spray, sublingual captopril or administration of intravenous labetalol.

Q8. Answer C

Chronic pelvic pain is a spectrum of conditions including urological, gynaecological, musculoskeletal and gastrointestinal pelvic pain syndromes. Urological syndromes comprising pelvic pain syndromes include prostate pain syndrome, bladder pain syndrome (including interstitial cystitis), genital pain syndrome and urethral pain syndrome.

Bladder pain syndrome is the preferred nomenclature for syndromes previously known as interstitial cystitis and painful bladder syndrome and this terminology has been adopted by the European Association of Urology and the International Association for the Study of Pain. Interstitial cystitis, described classically as the pathognomonic Hunner's ulcer and inflammation, is part of the spectrum of bladder pain syndrome.

A consensus criterion for the diagnosis of interstitial cystitis was developed following a series of workshops over 20 years ago. Interstitial cystitis is a symptom complex diagnosed by excluding known causes of symptoms. This NIDDK criteria was intended for use in scientific studies and is shown in Table 13.1:

Table 13.1 NIDDK diagnostic criteria for BPS/IC

Exclusion of IC/BPS	Inclusion criteria
Age <18 years	Pain on bladder filling relieved by voiding
Bladder tumour	Suprapubic, vaginal, pelvic, urethral or perineal pain
Radiation cystitis	Glomerulation on cystoscopy
Cystitis trabecula	Reduced bladder capacity on cystoscopy
Bacteria cystitis	Hunner's ulcers
Vaginitis	
Urethral diverticulum	
Genital ulcer	
Active herpes	
Stone disease	
Frequency <5 times	
Nocturia <2 times	
Duration <12 months	

Further Reading

Gillenwater JY, Wein AJ. Summary of the national institute of Arthritis, Diabetes, digestive and kidney diseases workshop on interstitial cystitis, national institutes of health, Bethesda, Maryland, August 28–29, 1987. *J Urol*, 1988; 140: 203–206.

Q9. Answer D

There are numerous treatment regimens for bladder pain syndrome with different modes of administration and mechanism of action. Oral therapy includes the histamine receptor antagonist hydroxyzine (blocking mast cell activation) and pentosan polysulphate (Elmiron) which acts by repairing defects in the GAG layer. Intravesical treatments include local anaesthetics, heparin, pentosan polysulphate, hyaluronic acid and dimethyl sulphoxide (DMSO). DMSO acts by scavenging free radicals thus decreasing inflammation. Hyaluronic acid acts by repairing defects in the GAG later and it is postulated that heparin has similarities with the GAG layer.

Further Reading

Vij M, Srikrishna S, Cardozo L. Interstitial cystitis: Diagnosis and management. *Eur Obstet Gynecol Reprod Biol*, 2012; 161: 1–7.

Q10. Answer B

The EPIC study (Irwin et al.) estimated the prevalence of lower urinary tract symptoms, overactive bladder, urinary incontinence and lower urinary tract symptoms suggestive of bladder outflow obstruction. Lower urinary tract symptoms were common, experienced by an estimated 45% of individuals, with a smaller proportion thought to be suggestive of bladder outflow obstruction (21.5%). Approximately 8% were estimated to suffer from urinary incontinence and 11% from overactive bladder symptoms.

Further Reading

Irwin DE, Zopp ZS, Agatep B, Milsom I, Abrams P. Worldwide prevalence estimates of lower urinary tract symptoms, overactive bladder, urinary incontinence and bladder outlet obstruction. *BJU Int*, 2011; 108(7): 1132–1138.

EMQs – ANSWERS

For the following clinical features listed below, what is the correct definition from the list above?

Q11. Answer M

Q12. Answer C

Q13. Answer B

Terminology for lower urinary tract symptoms has been standardised by the International Continence Society. Urgency is described as the complaint of a sudden compelling desire to pass urine which is difficult to defer. Increased daytime frequency is defined as the complaint by the patient that they void too often by day. Nocturia was defined in 2002 as the complaint that the individual has to wake at night once or more to void and it has to be preceded and followed by sleep. This has been updated in 2018 to the number of times urine is passed during the main sleep period. Having woken to pass urine for the first time, each urination must be followed by sleep or the intention to sleep. This should be quantified using a bladder diary.

Urinary incontinence is defined as the complaint of any loss of urine, and comprises stress (effort) incontinence, urgency urinary incontinence and mixed incontinence. Stress incontinence is the complaint of involuntary loss of urine on effort or on exertion, or on sneezing or coughing; urgency urinary incontinence is the complaint of involuntary leakage of urine accompanied by or immediately preceded by urgency and mixed urinary incontinence is the complaint of involuntary leakage of urine associated with urgency and also with exertion, effort, sneezing or coughing.

Further Reading

Abrams P, Cardozo L, Fall M, Griffiths D, Rosier P, Ulmsten U, et al. The standardisation of terminology of lower urinary tract function. Report from the Standardisation Sub-Committee of the ICS. *Neurourol Urodyn*, 2002; 21(2): 167–178.

Haylen BT, de Ridder D, Freeman RM, Swift SE, Berghmans B, Lee J, et al. International Urogynecological Association; International Continence Society. An International Urogynecological Association (IUGA)/International Continence Society (ICS) joint report on the terminology for female pelvic floor dysfunction. *Neurourol Urodyn*, 2010; 29(1): 4–20.

Hashim H, Blanker MH, Drake MJ, Djurhuus JC, Meijlink J, Morris V, et al. International continence society (ICS) report on the terminology for nocturia and nocturnal lower urinary tract function. *Neurourol Urodyn*, 2019; 38(2): 499–508.

Q14. Answer E

Q15. Answer G

Q16. Answer F

There are a number of pharmacological agents acting on the bladder. Anticholinergic medications, including solifenacin and fesoterodine, act on the muscarinic receptors with various subclass specificity. Broadly their efficacy of action is comparable, but the side effect profile varies according to the receptor specificity. Fesoterodine is a prodrug, converted to an active metabolite following administration. This active metabolite is the same as tolterodine but conversion is via a different mechanism which is theoretically faster.

Beta-3 agonists are another group of receptors present in the bladder and only one drug, Mirabegron, is commercially available as an oral agent for the treatment of overactive bladder. There is limited pharmacotherapy for the treatment of stress urinary incontinence; however, duloxetine is a serotonin noradrenaline reuptake inhibitor (SNRI) that can be used for women with moderate to severe stress urinary incontinence.

Capsaicin is an intravesical agent that blocks vanilloid receptors, blocking C-fibre afferent nerves leading to desensitisation, thus inhibiting detrusor contraction. Use is limited due to side effects of pain, but efficacy has been demonstrated in patients with neurogenic detrusor overactivity.

Desmopressin is used in the treatment of nocturia and nocturnal enuresis. It is a synthetic analogue of vasopressin and has an antidiuretic effect decreasing urine production at night.

Q17. Answer B

Q18. Answer C

Q19. Answer C

Pelvic organ prolapse may be assessed in two ways; the Halfway System (Baden & Walker) and the Pelvic Organ Prolapse Quantification System (POP-Q). The International Continence Society recommends use of the POP-Q.

The POP-Q uses a series or measurements using the hymen as a reference point to quantify the level of prolapse of the anterior vaginal wall, posterior vaginal wall and apex of the vagina. The results of these measurements are recorded in a grid along with additional measurements including total vaginal length, genital hiatus and perineal body. For the posterior vaginal wall, anterior vaginal wall and upper part of the vagina, two points are measured. Additional measurements of total vaginal length, perineal body and posterior fornix are also taken.

Aa	Ba	C
Anterior vaginal wall, 3 cm proximal to the hymen/introitus. This is a fixed point and usually corresponds to the urethrovesical junction. Range from −3 cm to +3 cm. Above or proximal to the hymen/introitus having a negative value and those below a positive value. 0 is at the level of the hymen/introitus.	Most distal (lowest) portion of remaining upper anterior vaginal wall.	Anterior vaginal fornix. Most distal edge of cervix or vaginal cuff.
Gh	**Pb**	**Tvl**
Genital hiatus: measured from the middle of the external urethral meatus to the posterior margin of the hymen/introitus.	Perineal body: measured from posterior margin of genital hiatus to the middle of the anal opening.	Total vaginal length: depth of vagina when points D & C are reduced to normal position.
Ap	**Bp**	**D**
Fixed point on the posterior vaginal wall, 3 cm proximal to hymen/introitus. Range as per Aa.	Most distal portion of the remaining upper posterior vaginal wall.	Posterior vaginal fornix.

Following assessment, prolapse is subsequently assigned by stage according to the most severe portion of the prolapse and also described by compartments (i.e., the anterior or posterior compartment and the cervix/vault).

Stage 0: No prolapse

Stage I: Most severe part of the prolapse is >1 cm proximal to hymen/introitus.

Stage II: Most severe part of the prolapse is within 1 cm either above or below the level of the hymen/introitus.

Stage III: Most severe part of the prolapse is >1 cm below the level of the hymen/introitus.

Stage IV: Almost complete eversion of the total length of the vagina (procidentia) (Figure 13.1A and 1B).

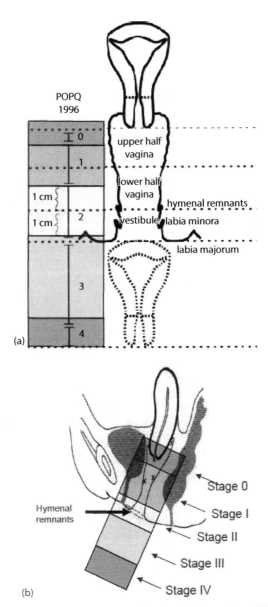

Figure 13.1 (a and b) Shows prolapse staging–0, I, II, III, IV (uterine by the position of the leading edge of the cervix).

Further Reading

Haylen BT, de Ridder D, Freeman RM, Swift SE, Berghmans B, Lee J, et al; International Urogynecological Association; International Continence Society. An International Urogynecological Association (IUGA)/International Continence Society (ICS) joint report on the terminology for female pelvic floor dysfunction. *Neurourol Urodyn*, 2010; 29(1): 4–20.

Q20. Answer C

Q21. Answer D

Q22. Answer A

There are numerous urological procedures that use bowel to either functionally augment the bladder, act as a conduit or replace the bladder orthotopically. A number of bowel segments can be used; however all methods are limited by complications. Metabolic complications differ according to which segment of bowel is used. When a segment of ileum is used in urinary diversion, hyperchloraemic metabolic acidosis may occur. This is due to the net absorption of ammonium and chloride ions from the urine, with secretion of sodium. Hyperchloraemic metabolic acidosis also occurs with the use of colonic segments. The use of stomach leads to hypochloraemic metabolic alkalosis accordingly. The use of jejunum leads to hyperkalaemic, hypochloraemic, hyponatraemic metabolic acidosis.

Q23. Answer E

Q24. Answer B

Q25. Answer C

Content/face validity relates to the assessment of whether the questionnaire makes sense to those being measured and to experts in the clinical area. Internal consistency (reliability) relates to the extent to which items within the questionnaire are related to each other. Stability (test-retest reliability) is the ability of whether the questionnaire measures the same sorts of things in the same person over a period of time. Construct validity relates to the relationships between the questionnaire and underlying theories. Criterion validity describes how well the questionnaire correlates with a 'gold standard' measure that already exists. Responsiveness measures change in questionnaires. Responsiveness indicates whether the measure can detect change in a patient's condition. An important aspect of responsiveness is determining not only whether the measure detects change but whether the change is meaningful to the patient. This can be done by determining the minimal important difference (MID) of the measure. The MID is the smallest change in a patient-reported outcome questionnaire score that would be considered meaningful or important to a patient.

CHAPTER 14: UROLOGICAL TRAUMA

Davendra M. Sharma, Sanjay Agarwal and Shyam Matanhelia

MCQs

Q1. What specific urological imaging investigation should be requested for a stable patient following blunt abdominal trauma who has dipstick haematuria?
A. CT KUB
B. IVU
C. Renal tract ultrasound
D. Contrast enhanced CT with 10 minute delayed scan
E. None of the above

Q2. What is the imaging investigation of choice in a stable patient with suspected renal trauma who has presented with visible haematuria?
A. Ultrasound renal tract
B. IVU
C. CT KUB
D. Contrast CT with delayed scan
E. None of the above

Q3. What is the difference between a Grade 3 and Grade 4 renal trauma injury?
A. Size of peri-renal haematoma
B. Depth of laceration
C. Contrast extravasation
D. Avulsion of the renal hilum
E. None of the above

Q4. When can penetrating injuries to the kidney be considered for non-operative management?
A. Knife entry point anterior to anterior axillary line in a stable patient
B. Gunshot injury to flank
C. Knife entry point posterior to anterior axillary line in a stable patient
D. Blast and fragment injury to flank
E. None of the above

Q5. When should main renal arterial injury be repaired, if suspected to be injured?
A. Within 24 hours
B. Within 18 hours
C. Within 12 hours
D. Within 6 hours
E. None of the above

Q6. In patients with renal trauma, immediate surgical exploration is required in which of the following scenarios?
A. Patients requiring blood transfusion
B. Grade 4 renal trauma
C. Bilateral high-grade renal trauma
D. Large peri-renal haematoma
E. None of the above

Q7. Which of the following principles are accepted standard practice in ureteric reconstruction after trauma?
A. Mobilisation of the ureter preserving the adventitia
B. Debridement of non-viable tissue
C. Spatulation of both ureteric ends
D. Tension-free anastomosis with fine absorbable sutures
E. All of the above

Q8. Which of the following is a strong indication for the surgical exploration of bladder trauma?
A. Recurrent catheter obstruction due to clots
B. Flame like contrast extravasation from the bladder
C. Haematuria following catheterisation
D. External fixation of an associated pelvic fracture
E. An associated urethral injury

Q9. In urethral trauma secondary to pelvic fracture, which of the following procedures is not used in the acute management?

A. Retrograde urethrogram
B. Antegrade urethrogram
C. Flexible urethroscopy
D. Ultrasound guided supra-pubic insertion of catheter
E. Gentle passage of a 14 F latex catheter

Q10. Suspected testicular rupture is best managed by:

A. Testicular exploration and repair
B. Bedrest, antibiotics and analgesia
C. MRI scanning
D. Testicular removal
E. Clinical examination – repeated if necessary.

Q11. A 24-year-old motorcyclist is brought into the Emergency department with a 'severe' pelvic fracture following a road traffic accident. Associated injuries mean that monitoring of urine output is required by the trauma team. What factor would immediately raise the suspicion of an associated urethral injury?

A. Blood at the meatus
B. Sleeve haematoma of penis
C. High riding prostate on digital rectal examination
D. Blood on glove following digital rectal examination
E. Butterfly haematoma of perineum

Q12. You are asked by the Gynaecology SPR to see a patient who had an abdominal hysterectomy 48 hours ago. The patient is tachycardic, pyrexial (39.2) and complaining of left flank pain. There is abdominal and left flank tenderness, and drainage of 500 mL of blood stained fluid in the last 12 hours from the pelvic drain. FBC – Hb 10.2, WCC 15.0. Electrolytes are normal. The next step in management is to:

A. Arrange urgent exploratory laparotomy and repair of suspected ureteric injury
B. Advise nil orally, bed rest, intravenous antibiotics and fluid replacement

C. Request urgent CT urogram after immediate resuscitation
D. Request urgent ultrasound
E. Arrange cystoscopy, retrograde ureteropyelogram and attempt retrograde JJ stenting

Q13. An 18-year-old male is brought in to the Emergency department after being stabbed in the right loin. There is no further history available. The patient's blood pressure is poorly maintained with intravenous fluids but stabilises with a 2 unit blood transfusion. Contrast CT shows a Grade 4 Right renal injury. There is no suspected intra-abdominal injury. What is the next step in management?

A. Request angioembolisation by experienced interventional radiologist
B. Urgent insertion of JJ stent
C. Urgent percutaneous drainage of peri-renal area
D. Admit for bed rest, regular observations and follow-up bloods.
E. Urgent exploratory laparotomy and kidney repair or nephrectomy

Q14. A 39-year-old male is brought to the Emergency Department complaining of severe lower abdominal pain and an inability to void. He had been involved in an altercation following a 'heavy' drinking session. He vaguely remembers being punched to the head and lower abdomen. He did not lose consciousness and has been assessed as having only a minor head injury. Examination reveals a stable patient with lower abdominal tenderness, but no obvious palpable bladder. Blood and urine tests are normal. What is the investigation would you consider next?

A. Intravenous urogram with delayed phase
B. Ascending urethrogram and insertion of catheter
C. Stress cystogram with 300 mL of contrast inserted into the bladder
D. Screening cystogram with diluted contrast
E. Ultrasound abdomen and renal tract

MCQs – ANSWERS

Q1. Answer E

Jack McAninch's data from the San Francisco General Hospital involved over 2000 patients with renal trauma at the time (1995) when it was recommended that stable patients with dipstick haematuria require no imaging. This was based on the findings that these patients very rarely had significant renal injuries and that in fact no significant injuries were missed in the non-imaged cohort of patients (1004). The accepted exception is a high index of suspicion of significant renal injury (e.g., fall from height and rapid deceleration injury). This is also supported by the EAU guidelines.

Q2. Answer D

The early phase of the contrast CT scan will delineate any vascular and parenchymal injuries. The 10-minute delayed scan will identify contrast extravasation.

Q3. Answer C

The accepted staging classification for renal trauma was developed by the American Association for Surgery of Trauma (AAST) Organ Injury Scaling Committee. It has been validated by several studies and it correlates well with the need for kidney repair or removal.

Q4. Answer C

Operative exploration has traditionally been recommended for penetrating injuries. However, if a knife entry point is posterior to the anterior axillary line, then the likelihood of renal hilar injury or associated visceral injury is low. High-resolution CT is leading to an increase in the non-operative management of this patient group. Low-velocity gunshot wounds can also be managed non-operatively.

Q5. Answer D

Renovascular injuries are uncommon. Renal salvage following main renal artery injury occurs in a quarter of patients at best. Time to reperfusion is the major factor in determining outcome and therefore expeditious intervention is required.

Q6. Answer E

Immediate surgical exploration is only required in patients with haemodynamic instability despite adequate resuscitation. Blood products can be used in the resuscitation phase and allow successful conservative management or angioembolisation. Grade 4 renal trauma should be managed without surgical intervention in the majority of cases. Bilateral injuries are a good indication for ultraconservative management, as the likelihood of nephrectomy increases dramatically with surgical intervention.

Q7. Answer E

Basic principles include all of these options as well as an internal ureteric stent and external drain.

Q8. Answer A

Flame like contrast extravasation suggests an extraperitoneal injury which can be managed conservatively. There is however, increasing data to support early surgical repair of extraperitoneal bladder injuries if internal fixation is performed. Catheter difficulties following bladder trauma are best managed by operative intervention and bladder repair.

Q9. Answer B

Antegrade urethrogram is useful in the planning of delayed reconstruction but is difficult and not helpful in the acute phase of management. Flexible urethroscopy can be used to assess the injury and catheterise the bladder per urethra.

Q10. Answer A

Urgent exploration should follow and will result in higher rates of testicular salvage.

Q11. Answer A

Blood at the meatus

Sleeve haematoma of penis – penile urethral injury (Buck's fascia intact)

High riding prostate on digital rectal examination (unreliable finding)

Blood on glove following digital rectal examination (rectal injury)

Butterfly haematoma of perineum (takes a while to develop)

Q12. Answer C

This patient has a urological injury until proven otherwise. It is essential to determine what injuries exist – right or left ureter, bladder or a combination. Contrast imaging is essential followed by nephrostomy in this sick patient. Once the patient is better, reconstruction can be considered.

Q13. Answer A

The so-called 'ultraconservative' approach to renal salvage should be followed in centres with the correct expertise. With the centralisation of trauma, these cases should not be managed in centres without 24 hours on call interventional radiology. Bleeding is the first priority and this should be controlled by selective angioembolisation. In the setting of urinary extravasation and penetrating trauma, embolisation should be followed by insertion of a ureteric stent. Unstable patients cannot be managed conservatively but operative intervention is likely to lead to nephrectomy.

Q14. Answer D

This patient's most likely diagnosis is an intraperitoneal bladder rupture from a direct blow to a full bladder. A stress cystogram is the investigation of choice in suspected bladder injuries. However intraperitoneal ruptures will lead to early contrast extravasation so neither the full volume (nor full strength contrast) should be used in these cases in the first instance.

CHAPTER 15: NEUROUROLOGY

Tina Rashid and Rizwan Hamid

MCQs

Q1. In autonomic dysreflexia, which of the following symptoms do patients typically experience?
- A. Flushing above the level of the injury, hypertension, reflex bradycardia and headache
- B. Flushing above the level of the injury, hypertension, reflex tachycardia and headache
- C. Flushing below the level of the injury, hypotension, reflex bradycardia and headache
- D. Flushing below the level of the injury, hypertension, reflex tachycardia and headache
- E. Flushing below the level of the injury, hypertension, reflex brachycardia and headache

Q2. An upper motor neurone lesion will usually comprise which of the following features?
- A. A lesion at T10 or above with an atonic bladder
- B. A lesion at T10 or above with neurogenic detrusor overactivity and detrusor-sphincter-dyssynergia
- C. A lesion below L2 with an atonic bladder
- D. Any lesion with detrusor-sphincter-dyssynergia
- E. Cauda equina compression

Q3. When considering metabolic changes in substitution cystoplasties using bowel, which of the following is CORRECT?
- A. A mild, subclinical hyperchloremic metabolic acidosis is encountered in *all* patients that undergo urinary diversion using ileal and/or colonic segments.
- B. Resulting hypokalaemia can lead to Guillain-Barré syndrome.
- C. Hypochloraemic hyperkalaemic metabolic acidosis is common.
- D. Follow-up of such patients is required for up to 10 years after their initial surgery.
- E. Is more common in a conduit than in a reservoir reconstruction.

Q4. Which of the following is TRUE in spinal shock?
- A. Is defined as a spinal cord concussion associated with paralysis, hypotonia and hyperreflexia.
- B. Usually lasts for 3 days.
- C. Ends when the bulbocavernosus reflex returns.
- D. The bladder should only be managed by CISC.
- E. Is more common in women.

Q5. Which of the following is TRUE regarding onabotulinum toxin A?
- A. Was first used in urological terms for treatment of neurogenic detrusor overactivity
- B. Is a temporary treatment and requires re-injections for sustained benefit
- C. Takes effect immediately
- D. Selectively inhibits post-synaptic vesicular acetylcholine release by cleaving SNAP-25
- E. Is not licensed for patients with idiopathic detrusor overactivity

Q6. Which is CORRECT for the artificial urinary sphincter (AUS)?
- A. It is the method of choice to treat stress urinary incontinence secondary to neurogenic bladder dysfunction.
- B. In a patient with neuropathic bladder, the cuff should be placed at the bulbar

urethral sphincter in a man and at the bladder neck in a woman.

C. It must not be placed at the same time as a 'clam' cystoplasty due to the risk of device infection.

D. The revision rate is equivalent in neuropaths and non-neuropaths.

E. The infection rate is 10%.

Q7. **Which of the following statements is CORRECT with respect to sacral anterior root stimulator (SARS)?**

A. At the time of implantation, it is usual to perform a concurrent dorsal rhizotomy, which involves dividing the posterior roots of S2 and S3.

B. Should be accompanied by dorsal rhizotomy in patients with both complete and incomplete spinal cord lesions.

C. The benefits include increased bladder capacity and compliance.

D. Causes reflex erection in a man.

E. May cause constipation.

Q8. **Which is TRUE regarding anticholinergic medications?**

A. Oxybutynin causes direct smooth muscle relaxation via calcium channel blockade.

B. Tolterodine is M3 receptor specific.

C. M3 receptors are more abundant in the detrusor but M2 receptors are functionally more important.

D. The STAR study compared efficacy, side effect profile and discontinuation rates of solifenacin 5 mg with 10 mg.

E. Fesoterodine is a prodrug that after oral administration is hydrolysed to the same active metabolite as oxybutynin.

Q9. **Which is CORRECT regarding neuroanatomy of the bladder?**

A. Parasympathetic nerves arise from T10-L2.

B. Sympathetic nerves arise from T11-L2.

C. Somatic nerves arise from L2-L4.

D. Pudendal nerve has fibres that originate from Onuf's nucleus at the medial border of anterior horn.

E. All of the above.

Q10. **The urodynamic trace below demonstrates the following feature:**

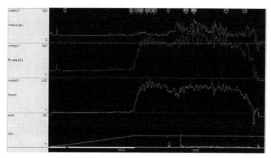

A. The voiding phase is normal.

B. There are no cough tests on this trace.

C. The abdominal line is not functioning well.

D. Classical sawtooth appearance of neurogenic detrusor overactivity with sustained high pressure contraction.

E. More than 500 mL have been instilled.

MCQs – ANSWERS

Q1. Answer A

Autonomic dysreflexia is a life-threatening emergency which can occur in patients with spinal cord injuries (SCI) at or above T6. There is massive sympathetic discharge of the distal autonomous cord (i.e., below the level of the spinal cord injury) secondary to specific stimulus. Ordinarily the reflexes would be inhibited by output from the medulla but in SCI this does not happen and leads to autonomic dysreflexia.

The most common cause is bladder distension due to a blocked catheter, cystoscopy or urodynamics. Other causes include faecal loading, skin, and urine infections. Symptoms are flushing and sweating of skin above the level of injury, hypertension with reflex bradycardia and headache. The crucial step is to identify it, remove the offending stimulus, sit the patient up and administer 10 mg nifedipine to chew, not sublingually. Blood pressure must be monitored throughout [1].

Q2. Answer B

In spinal cord injuries at or above the level of T10, the patient is most likely to have an upper motor neurone type injury with neurogenic detrusor overactivity and detrusor-sphincter-dyssynergia (DSD). DSD is defined as involuntary contraction of the urethral and/or periure-thral striated muscle simultaneously with a detrusor contraction. This is the result of loss of co-ordination by the pontine micturition centre. The typical appearance on a pressure-flow trace is drawn as shown in Figure 15.1.

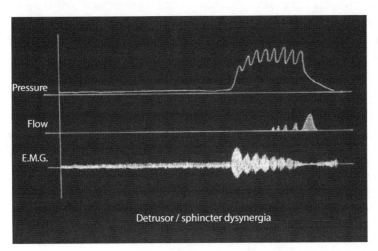

Figure 15.1 Pressure/flow trace and EMG in a spinal cord injured patient with DSD. (From Hussain, M. et al., *BJMSU*, 5, 192–203, 2012.)

Q3. Answer A

In the bowel lumen, sodium ions (Na^+) are secreted in exchange for hydrogen ions (H^+) and bicarbonate ions (HCO_3^-) in exchange for chloride ions (Cl^-).

Urine has high concentrations of ammonia (NH_3), ammonium (NH_4^+), hydrogen and chloride – these substances are reabsorbed in bowel segments exposed to urine resulting in chronic acid load. Whether this results in significant metabolic acidosis depends on the patient (comorbidities), bowel segment used and the duration of contact of the bowel with urine.

A mild, subclinical hyperchloremic metabolic acidosis is encountered in *all* patients that undergo urinary diversion using bowel. ≤20% of these will have episodes of severe acidosis. 10% of patients with an ileal conduit have a clinically important metabolic acidosis after 1 year [2,3].

Renal wasting and secretion of potassium from the bowel results in hypokalaemia. In general, this will not have important clinical consequences. However, when metabolic acidosis is treated, potassium is exchanged with the intracellular space causing further potassium depletion, manifesting clinically as muscle weakness. Several cases of muscle weakness mistaken for Guillain-Barré syndrome after ureterosigmoidostomy are reported [4–6]. Therefore, when correcting acidosis also supplement potassium (potassium citrate 15 mEq or 1.6 g BD-QDS) [7].

Lifelong follow-up of patients with bowel substitutions is recommended, comprising bloods (FBC, U&E, bicarbonate, chloride, B12, folate) and USS KUB at regular intervals.

Q4. Answer C

Spinal shock involves a spinal cord concussion, which usually involves a period of paralysis, hypotonia and areflexia. All reflex activity below the level of the lesion is abated. At its conclusion there may be hyperreflexia, hypertonicity and clonus. It can last for up to 12 weeks, but the time period is variable. Return of reflex activity below the level of injury indicates the end of spinal shock.

The bulbocavernosus reflex (anal sphincter contraction in response to squeezing the glans penis or tugging on the urethral catheter) involves the S2, S3 nerve roots and is a spinal cord mediated reflex. Initial management of spinal shock involves urethral catheterisation with the aim of converting the patient over to intermittent catheterisation (self or by carer) as soon as possible.

Be careful not to mix up spinal shock and autonomic dysreflexia.

Q5. Answer B

Onabotulinum toxin A was first used in 1988 for the treatment of detrusor-sphincter dyssynergia. The first report for neurogenic detrusor overactivity was by Schurch in 2000. It is a selective inhibitor of *presynaptic* vesicular acetylcholine release by cleaving the synaptosomal-associated protein 25 (SNAP-25). The effects are temporary lasting on an average of 6–9 months. Re-injections are equally effective. It is generally performed under local anaesthesia with a flexible cystoscope as a day case procedure. Whilst originally licensed in the UK for use in neurogenic detrusor overactivity, in 2019 it was licensed for use in idiopathic detrusor overactivity (NICE).

Q6. Answer A

The bulbar urethra is the preferred cuff implantation site in post-prostatectomy incontinence. In neuropaths, in particular after spinal cord injury, patients are mostly wheelchair bound thus sitting with the whole-body weight on the bulbar urethra. Moreover, neuropathic patients often have an open bladder neck, especially in patients with infrasacral lesions. Consequently, the prostatic urethra is always filled with urine, which may possibly be a factor for recurrent infection and prostatic influx in male patients. Therefore, in neuropaths, the AUS cuff is placed at the bladder neck. The infection rate is 1%–5%. In non-neuropaths, the erosion rate is also 1%–5% but is higher in neuropaths. It is possible to place an artificial urinary sphincter at the same time whilst performing a cystoplasty. However, there can be an increased risk of infection and the patient must be warned accordingly.

Q7. Answer A

SARS is also known as the Brindley or Finetech-Brindley stimulator. The sacral anterior root stimulator was developed by experiments on baboons in the MRC Neurological Prostheses Unit in London from 1969 to 1977 [8].

Activation of the implant stimulates contraction of both the bladder and the external sphincter. However, because the bladder is composed of smooth muscle and the sphincter-striated muscle, sphincter contraction is relatively short, and the detrusor continues to contract (and therefore empty) long after sphincter contraction is complete. This improves bladder emptying, reduces residual volume and infection and lowers transmitted upper tract pressures. The posterior roots are cut to control neurogenic overactivity. The improvement in bladder capacity and compliance is secondary to the dorsal rhizotomy and not the SARS.

The effects of implant activation on the bowel are increased colonic activity, reduced constipation and sometimes defaecation during stimulation. Dorsal rhizotomy causes loss of reflex erection but activation of the implant will cause a penile erection.

Q8. Answer A

M2 receptors are more abundant in the detrusor but M3 receptors are functionally more important. Anticholinergics work at muscarinic receptors to reduce the response to cholinergic stimulation, thus reducing detrusor contractions and detrusor pressure during filling.

Oxybutynin has some selectivity for M1 and M3 receptor subtypes as well as direct smooth muscle relaxant affect, probably via calcium channel blockade. Randomised trials have confirmed the efficacy of oxybutynin at the expense of compliance due to side effect profiles. ER oxybutynin has comparable efficacy to immediate release but improved tolerability [9].

Tolterodine is not receptor specific but has greater affinity for the bladder compared to other organs. IR tolterodine has equivalent efficacy to oxybutynin with fewer side effects.

Solifenacin is an M3 receptor antagonist. The STAR trial [10] was a prospective, double-blind, 12-week study to compare efficacy and safety of solifenacin 5 or 10 mg and tolterodine ER 4 mg once daily in OAB patients. The study concluded that solifenacin had greater efficacy in decreasing urgency episodes, incontinence, urgency incontinence and pad usage and increasing the volume voided per micturition. Discontinuations were comparable and low in both groups.

Fesoterodine is a prodrug that is hydrolysed to the same active metabolite as tolterodine.

[ER] = extended release; [IR] = immediate release; [OAB] = overactive bladder

Q9. Answer B

The "wiring" of the bladder consists of an excitatory input by efferent parasympathetic nerves originating in the S_2–S_4 intermediolateral columns of the spinal cord.

The sympathetic input to the bladder arises from neurons originating from the intermediolateral column of the T_{11}–L_2 spinal cord segments, in order to innervate the trigone and bladder neck smooth muscle.

The lower urinary tract is innervated by three types of peripheral nerves: parasympathetic (cholinergic) nerves, sympathetic (noradrenergic) nerves and somatic (cholinergic) nerves. The lateral border of the ventral horn (Onuf's nucleus) is the origin of the cholinergic motor neurones to the external urethral sphincter. Fibres travel via the pudendal nerves (S_2 and S_3) to contract this sphincter.

Q10. Answer D

The safety of the patient should be paramount during the study. There should be careful assessment of the patient's ability to sit and stand safely and this should be documented in the report. The investigator should understand the phenomenon of autonomic dysreflexia (AD) and be competent to treat this life-threatening condition.

It is recommended to start filling at 20 mL/min with body warm fluid. This trace demonstrates a classical pattern of neurogenic detrusor overactivity and if accompanied with a video clip would have shown sphincter dyssynergia. There is a cough test in the beginning of the study with good subtraction. Ideally, the cough should be performed after every minute and at the end of the study to ensure optimal functioning of the lines. Although not clearly marked, it is unlikely more than 500 mL has been instilled in the bladder.

REFERENCES

1. Hussain, M., J. Shah, R. Hamid, Neurourology: A review. *BJMSU*, 2012, 5: 192–203.
2. Shimko, M.S., M.K. Tollefson, E.C. Umbreit et al., Long-term complications of conduit urinary diversion. *J Urol*, 2011, 185(2): 562–567.
3. McDougal, W.A.K., M.O. Koch, Impaired growth and development and urinary intestinal interposition. *Abst Am Assoc GU Surg*, 1991, 105: 3.
4. Valtier, B., G. Mion, L.H. Pham et al., Severe hypokalaemic paralysis from an unusual cause mimicking the Guillain-Barre syndrome. *Intensive Care Med*, 1989, 15(8): 534–535.
5. Van Bekkum, J.W., D.J. Bac, I.E. Nienhuis et al., Life-threatening hypokalaemia and quadriparesis in a patient with ureterosigmoidostomy. *Neth J Med*, 2002, 60(1): 26–28.
6. Rafique, M., Life threatening hypokalemia and quadriparesis in a patient with ureterosigmoidostomy. *Int Urol Nephrol*, 2006, 38(3–4): 453–456.
7. Bersch, U., K. Göcking, J. Pannek., The artificial urinary sphincter in patients with spinal cord lesion: Description of a modified technique and clinical results. *Eur Urol*, 2009, 55: 687–695.
8. Brindley, G.S., The first 500 patients with sacral anterior root stimulator implants: General description. *Paraplegia*, 1994, 32(12): 795–805.
9. Anderson, R.U., Mobley, D., Blank, B., Saltzstein, D., Susset, J., Brown, J.S., Once daily controlled versus immediate release oxybutynin chloride for urge urinary incontinence. OROS Oxybutynin Study Group. *J Urol* 1999, 161(6): 1809–1812.
10. Chapple, C.R., R. Martinez-Garcia, L. Selvaggi, P. Toozs-Hobson, W. Warnack, T. Drogendijk, D.M. Wright, J. Bolodeoku, STAR study group. A comparison of the efficacy and tolerability of solifenacin succinate and extended release tolterodine at treating overactive bladder syndrome: Results of the STAR trial. *Eur Urol* 2005, 48(3): 464–470.

CHAPTER 16: UROLITHIASIS

Thomas Johnston, James Armitage and Oliver Wiseman

MCQs

Q1. The following are true of renal calculi in pregnancy, except:
A. Pregnancy is an absolute contraindication to ureteroscopic stone removal.
B. Pregnancy is an absolute contraindication to extracorporeal shockwave lithotripsy.
C. Stent insertion may be preferred under local anaesthesia.
D. Hypercalciuria of pregnancy typically necessitates frequent changes of ureteric stent/percutaneous nephrostomy tubes where conservative management has failed.
E. Conservative management results in the spontaneous passage of stones in 60%–80%.

Q2. The following are recognised inhibitors of stone formation in the metastable zone except:
A. Tamm-Horsfall protein
B. Citrate
C. Nephrocalcin
D. Uropontin
E. Oxalate

Q3. Urease producing organisms include all of the following, except:
A. *Staphylococcus aureus*
B. *Escherichia coli*
C. *Ureaplasma urealyticum*
D. *Proteus mirabilis*
E. *Helicobacter pylori*

Q4. The following represent unfavourable characteristics for successful extracorporeal shockwave lithotripsy to a lower pole stone except:
A. Infundibulopelvic angle <90 degrees
B. Calcium oxalate dihydrate stone
C. Calcium oxalate monohydrate stone
D. Cystine stones
E. Obesity (skin to stone distance >10 cm)

Q5. The following dietary advice should be given to a first time calcium oxalate stone former with normal serum calcium and a normal 24-hour urine collection except:
A. Maintain a fluid intake of between 2.5–3.0 L/day
B. Aim to pass 2.0–2.5 L/day urine
C. Restrict calcium intake to under 1000 mg/day
D. Avoid excess salt in the diet (max. 3–5 g/day)
E. Limit protein intake to 0.8–1.0 g/kg/day

Q6. Which of the following is true regarding extracorporeal shockwave lithotripsy?
A. ESWL is more effective than ureteroscopy for an 8-mm distal ureteric stone.
B. Anticoagulation with warfarin is not an absolute contraindication.
C. Hounsfield Units (HU) of the stone is of limited use in predicting success.
D. Fragmentation is more successful at a shock rate of 1 Hz compared to 2 Hz.
E. Shockwaves converge on focal point F1 where stone fragmentation occurs.

Q7. The following are true of stones in horseshoe kidneys except:
A. PUJ obstruction and abnormal drainage of horseshoe kidneys predisposes to urinary stasis and stone formation in approximately 20%.
B. Horseshoe kidneys are malrotated such that their calyces are situated in a medial position.

C. The blood supply is quite variable and may predispose to increased bleeding risk with PCNL.

D. Extracorporeal shockwave lithotripsy is contraindicated.

E. The use of flexible nephroscopes and flexible ureteroscopes may reduce the need for multiple punctures where PCNL is used to treat stones in horseshoe kidneys.

Q8. **The following are true of cystinuria, except:**

A. Cystinuria is inherited as an autosomal dominant condition with an incidence of 1 in 20,000.

B. The pKa of cystine is 8.3 and the cyanide nitroprusside test is used to test for cystinuria.

C. Treatment with effervescent ascorbic acid (vitamin C) may increase the solubility of cystine.

D. Homozygous cystinurics typically pass more than 600-mg cystine in their urine per day.

E. Cystine stones are usually visible on plain abdominal radiograph due to the presence of disulphide bonds.

Q9. **The following are true of bladder calculi, except:**

A. In the Western world bladder calculi are most commonly composed of uric acid.

B. Malnutrition and low phosphate diets predispose to endemic bladder stones in the developing world.

C. More than 90% of men with bladder calculi require surgery for bladder outflow obstruction.

D. Cystolitholopaxy should be undertaken before bladder outflow surgery where the procedures are combined.

E. The holmium laser may be used to treat large bladder calculi as an alternative to open stone removal.

Q10. **The following are true regarding analgesia in patients presenting with acute ureteric colic, except:**

A. Non-steroidal anti-inflammatory drugs (NSAIDs) are associated with less vomiting than opioids.

B. NSAIDs have been shown to reduce glomerular filtration rate and intrarenal pressure through their action on prostaglandin synthesis.

C. Less 'rescue' medication is required with NSAIDs compared to opioids.

D. Analgesia should not be given until a firm diagnosis of ureteric colic has been made to prevent diagnostic confusion.

E. Rectal administration of NSAIDs should be considered, especially in patients who present with vomiting.

Q11. **Regarding flexible ureteroscopes the following is true:**

A. They are routinely used in the treatment of patients with lower ureteric stones.

B. Of single-use flexible ureteroscopes, only the fibre-optic variety are currently available.

C. The working channel is usually 2.8 F.

D. Digital scopes may limit access to the kidney due to their larger tip size.

E. The maximum deflection available is 180°–180°.

Q12. **The following are acceptable first-line treatments for a 1.5 cm renal pelvic stone in a patient with a normal contralateral kidney, except:**

A. ESWL

B. Flexible ureteroscopy with stent insertion

C. Flexible ureteroscopy without stent insertion

D. PCNL

E. Laparoscopic or open pyelolithotomy

Q13. **The following are true of non-metallic ureteric stents, except:**

A. They may encrust within a few weeks in patients with cystinuria and in pregnancy.

B. They may be inserted to relieve obstruction in patients with pyonephrosis secondary to a proximal ureteric stone.

C. Complications include encrustation and ureteric reflux.

D. Indwell time should not exceed six months.

E. Alpha-blocker medication has been shown to reduce stent symptoms.

Q14. Enteric (secondary) hyperoxaluria can occur as a result of the following, except:
A. Insufficient dietary calcium intake
B. Intake of high doses of ascorbic acid
C. Increased occurrence of oxalate-degrading bacteria such as *Oxalobacter formigenes*
D. Inflammatory bowel disease
E. Intoxication with ethylene glycol

Q15. The following are true of extracorporeal shock wave lithotriptors, except:
A. The Dornier HM1 lithotriptor, developed in 1980, was the first lithotripter to be used to treat renal calculi in vivo.
B. The Stortz Modulith® is an example of a electromagnetic lithotripter, where magnetic energy is applied to crystals to generate the shockwave.
C. Electrohydraulic lithotriptors often incorporate an angulated hemispherical dish to focus shock waves created by an underwater spark gap.
D. Piezoelectric lithotriptors utilise multiple ceramic crystals arranged around a hemispherical dish.
E. The Dornier HM3 lithotriptor, the first commercial device, required immersion of the fully anaesthetised patient in a water bath.

Q16. The following are true for renal tubular acidosis (RTA) except:
A. Type 1 RTA is the failure of H^+ secretion in the distal nephron tubules.
B. Type 1 RTA is the failure of H^+ secretion is characterised by hyperchloraemic metabolic acidosis (normal anion gap).
C. Type 1 RTA typically form calcium phosphate stones.

D. Treatment of distal RTA should not be undertaken with potassium citrate, which has the effect of increasing urine pH.
E. The ammonium chloride acidification test with a urinary pH > 5.5 being indicative of RTA.

Q17. The following are true of hypercalciuria and its relation to stone formation, except:
A. It is often associated with calcium oxalate dihydrate stones.
B. Can be treated with a thiazide diuretic.
C. Is defined as the excretion of >5.5 mmol/24 hours of urinary calcium in a male.
D. Can be associated with excessive salt intake.
E. Can arise as a result of primary hyperparathyroidism.

Q18. Which of the following is the most important factor in uric acid stone formation?
A. Low urinary pH
B. High urinary pH
C. Hyperuricaemia
D. Hyperuricosuria
E. Low oral intake

Q19. The following antibiotics are safe in one *or* all trimesters of pregnancy, except:
A. Co-amoxiclav
B. Trimethoprim
C. Nitrofurantoin
D. Cefalexin
E. Gentamicin

Q20. The most common type of urinary stone is:
A. Calcium oxalate
B. Calcium phosphate
C. Uric acid
D. Infection
E. Cystine

EMQs

Q21–27. Treatment options for urinary tract stones
  A. Observation
  B. Medical expulsive therapy (according to EAU guidelines)
  C. Extracorporeal shockwave lithotripsy
  D. Primary ureteroscopic stone removal
  E. Percutaneous nephrolithotomy
  F. Ureteric stent
  G. Urinary alkalinisation
  H. Percutaneous nephrostomy
  I. Open stone removal
  J. Laparoscopic stone removal
  K. Nephrectomy

Please select the most appropriate first-line treatment option, from the list above, for each of the clinical scenarios, listed below.

Q21. A 7-mm stone at the vesicoureteric junction stone in a patient who is clinically well and whose pain is well controlled.

Q22. A 5-mm stone in a lower pole calyx identified as an incidental finding in a 76-year-old patient who is asymptomatic.

Q23. A 66-year-old lady with a complete staghorn calculus in a poorly functioning kidney (9%). She has no comorbidity and is asymptomatic other than occasional urinary tract infections.

Q24. A 1-cm radio-opaque stone at the pelvic-ureteric junction. The patient presented with loin pain but is now pain-free, has normal renal function and exhibits no signs of sepsis.

Q25. A 7-mm mid-ureteric stone in a 36/40 pregnant woman who is clinically well without complicating features.

Q26. An 8-mm proximal ureteric stone, visible on plain film, without complicating features.

Q27. A 3-cm lower pole partial staghorn stone in a patient with equal differential renal function.

Q28–32. Urinary stones metaphylaxis
  A. Urinary alkalinisation to pH > 6.5 and increase fluid intake
  B. Urinary alkalinisation to pH > 7.5 and increase fluid intake
  C. Urinary acidification and increase fluid intake
  D. D-Penicillamine and increase fluid intake
  E. L-methionine and increase fluid intake
  F. Thiazide diuretic and increase fluid intake
  G. Increase fluid intake only
  H. Alkaline citrate plus allopurinol and increase fluid intake

Please select the most appropriate means of metaphylaxis from the list above, in addition to increased fluid intake, for each of the following clinical scenarios described below.

Q28. A 22-year-old woman who presents for the first time with a cystine stone treated successfully with PCNL. She is now stone free.

Q29. A 43-year-old man who had ureteroscopy for a calcium oxalate stone. The sole abnormality on 24 hours urine collection is hyperuricosuria.

Q30. A 35-year-old man who passed a 5 mm uric acid stone. He has normal serum and urinary urate. 24 hours urine collection shows a urinary volume of 3 L/day.

Q31. A recurrent calcium oxalate stone former with hypercalciuria on 24 hours urine collection (>10 mmol/day). Parathyroid hormone levels are normal.

Q32. Recurrent calcium oxalate stone former. Urine volume 0.8 L/day and full metabolic screen otherwise normal.

Q33–38. Biochemistry of kidney stones
  A. Calcium oxalate
  B. Calcium phosphate
  C. Uric acid

D. Cystine

E. Struvite

F. Not at increased risk of stones

For each of the following clinical conditions listed below, please choose the most commonly associated type of kidney stone, from the list above.

Q33. Inflammatory bowel disease

Q34. Hyperparathyroidism

Q35. Type 1 (distal or complete) renal tubular acidosis

Q36. Type 2 (proximal or incomplete) renal tubular acidosis

Q37. Gout

Q38. Recurrent urinary tract infections

Q39–43. Endourology retrieval devices
  A. 1.9 Fr tipless basket
  B. Stainless steel flat wire basket (e.g., Segura®)
  C. Tri-radiate graspers
  D. Anti-retropulsion device (e.g., Stone cone®, Entrap®)
  E. Ureteroscopic biopsy forceps

For each of the following clinical scenario at ureteroscopy listed below, choose the most appropriate retrieval device, from the options above.

Q39. Retrieval of small stone fragments from the kidney

Q40. Attempted removal of an intact 4-mm distal ureteric stone

Q41. Removal of a large pedunculated ureteric polyp intact

Q42. During fragmentation of a 1-cm proximal ureteric stone, if no flexible ureteroscope available

Q43. Biopsy of a flat ureteric lesion

Q44–50. Holmium laser fibre settings
  A. 200 μm laser fibre on setting 0.4 J 20 Hz, long pulse width
  B. 200 μm laser fibre on setting 0.4 J 20 Hz, short pulse width
  C. 200 μm laser fibre on setting 1.4 J 8 Hz, long pulse width
  D. 550 μm laser fibre on setting 1 J 30 Hz
  E. 200 μm laser fibre on setting 1 J 10 Hz, long pulse width
  F. 550 μm laser fibre on setting 2 J 50 Hz
  G. 200 μm laser fibre on setting 1.4 J 8 Hz, short pulse width
  H. 365 μm laser fibre on setting 0.4 J 20 Hz, long pulse width

Which of the above are the most appropriate holmium laser fibre and initial setting for each clinical scenario listed below?

Q44. Semi-rigid ureteroscopic fragmentation and extraction of an 8-mm distal ureteric stone

Q45. Fragmentation of a large bladder stone

Q46. Ureteroscopic dusting of a 6-mm lower pole renal stone

Q47. Ureteroscopic fragmentation and extraction of large stone fragments in the upper pole

Q48. Proximal ureteric urothelial carcinoma treatment

Q49. Incision of pelviureteric junction

Q50. Holmium laser enucleation of prostate

Q51–57. Side effects of medical treatment for urolithiasis
  A. Dry cough
  B. Hypercalciuria
  C. Glucose intolerance
  D. Diarrhoea and gastrointestinal symptoms
  E. Hyperoxaluria

For the following medical treatments to prevent stone recurrence, please choose the most commonly associated side effect from the list above.

Q51. Bendroflumethiazide

Q52. Ascorbic acid

Q53. Captopril

Q54. Sodium bicarbonate

Q55. D-Penicillamine

Q56. Thiola

Q57. Potassium citrate

Q58–61. Guidewires
A. 150-cm long, nitinol core, PTFE coating, hydrophilic tip
B. 150-cm long, nitinol core, PTFE coating, hydrophobic tip
C. 300-cm long, stainless steel core, PTFE coating
D. 150-cm long, stainless steel core, PTFE coating, hydrophilic tip
E. 150-cm long, stainless steel core, PTFE coating
F. 150-cm long, nitinol core, hydrophilic coating
G. 150-cm long, stainless steel core, hydrophilic coating

For each of the following guidewires, please chose the most accurate description, from the list above.

Q58. Amplatz® super stiff

Q59. Terumo®

Q60. Benston/PTFE wire

Q61. Sensor®

Q62–68. Mechanism of action of common antibiotics used in clinical practice
A. Inhibits dihydrofolate reductase
B. Prevents peptidoglycan bacterial cell wall formation
C. Inhibit bacterial protein synthesis (bind to ribosomal subunit 50 S and target 23 S ribosomal RNA)
D. Inhibits DNA gyrase therefore prevents transcription or replication
E. Inhibit bacterial protein synthesis (inhibit ribosomes)

For each of the following antibiotics, please chose the most appropriate mechanism of action from the list above.

Q62. Trimethoprin

Q63. Nitrofurantoin

Q64. Ciprofloxacin

Q65. Co-amoxiclav

Q66. Cephalexin

Q67. Gentamicin

Q68. Meropenem

Q69–74. Morphology of kidney stones crystals during urine light microscopy:
A. Calcium oxalate monohydrate
B. Uric acid
C. Cystine
D. Struvite
E. Calcium oxalate dihydrate
F. Calcium phosphate

For each of the following kidney stone crystals shapes please chose the corresponding kidney stone type, from the list above.

Q69. Hexagonal

Q70. Coffin-lid

Q71. Envelope

Q72. Dumbbell

Q73. Flat shaped or wedge prisms

Q74. Needle shaped

MCQs – ANSWERS

Q1. Answer A

The incidence of urolithiasis in pregnancy is similar to that in non-pregnant women because a greater concentration of inhibitors of stone formation such as citrate, magnesium and glycosaminoglycans counter the effects of hypercalcaemia, hypercalciuria and urinary stasis. Pregnant women with symptoms suggestive of acute ureteric colic are best investigated initially by ultrasound particularly in the first trimester where radiation risks (teratogenesis, carcinogenesis and mutagenesis) are greatest. However, it may be difficult to differentiate acute ureteric obstruction from the physiological hydronephrosis that is often seen on the right side in pregnancy. Transvaginal ultrasound can be helpful to assess the distal ureter. MRI is advised as a second line investigation when results are equivocal and is able to define the level of urinary obstruction, visualise stones as a filling defect and can assess non-urological organ systems. Low-dose non-contrast CT KUB (foetal exposure 0.05 Gy versus 2.5 Gy) is increasing in popularity with a high sensitivity and specificity but still is last-line as exposure to ionising radiation can be associated with teratogenic risks and development of childhood malignancies.

Conservative management is the preferred treatment option for pregnant women with ureteric stones as the majority will pass spontaneously [1]. This may be the result of ureteral dilatation secondary to the effects of elevated levels of circulating progesterone. Where expectant management fails or intervention is indicated on the grounds of infection or in the presence of a solitary kidney, urinary diversion with a percutaneous nephrostomy or ureteric stent should be considered next. This usually leads to the rapid relief of symptoms but may necessitate frequent (up to six weekly) nephrostomy or stent changes because hypercalciuria leads to rapid encrustation.

Ureteroscopy has been shown to be effective and safe in pregnancy with complication rates similar to those observed in non-pregnant women [2]. On the other hand, pregnancy is considered an absolute contraindication to extracorporeal shockwave lithotripsy (ESWL) following studies on mice that demonstrated foetal damage and death in the later stages of pregnancy [3].

Q2. Answer E

Stone formation depends on the concentration of precipitating substances in urine and reflects a complex relationship between factors that can be categorised into either promoters of crystallisation or inhibitors of crystal formation and aggregation (see Figure 16.1) [4].

Urine is ordinarily supersaturated with calcium oxalate and may be supersaturated with other compounds such as calcium phosphate and sodium and ammonium urate. However, supersaturation is variable and in the metastable zone crystal aggregation will not occur unless induced by epitaxy (one salt inducing the precipitation of another salt) or heterogenous nucleation caused by the influence of foreign particles; for example, bacteria acting as niduses for stone formation.

Crystals of one salt have been shown to induce the precipitation of crystals of other salts by a process referred to as epitaxy. For example, calcium phosphate or calcium carbonate crystals may stimulate precipitation of calcium oxalate crystals and thereby promote stone formation.

It is believed that the presence of endogenous compounds such as magnesium, zinc, fluoride and citrate act as inhibitors of stone crystallisation and are the reason that stones do not generally form in urine despite its supersaturation.

Tamm-Horsfall protein, also known as uromodulin, is produced by the thick ascending limb of the loop of Henle. Its role in urolithiasis remains uncertain but it may act as both a promoter and inhibitor of stone formation. Uropontin and nephrocalcin are also glycoproteins that are thought to have an effect on kidney stone formation.

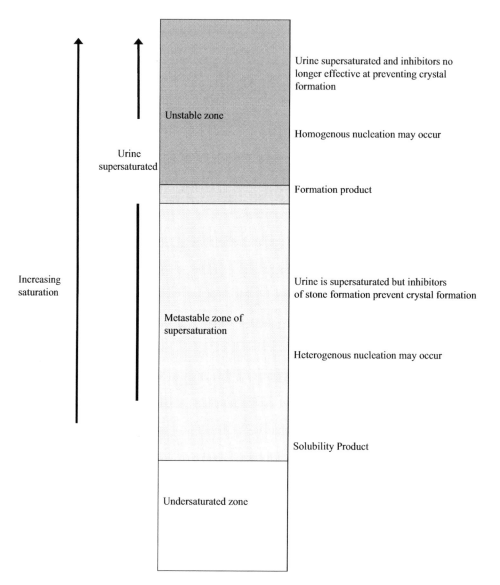

Figure 16.1   Relationship between urinary saturation and promoters and inhibitors of stone formation.

Q3. Answer B

Urease is an enzyme that is produced by many Gram-negative, Gram-positive and Mycoplasma bacteria. *Proteus* species, *Klebsiella* species and *Pseudomonas aeruginosa* are examples of Gram-negative urease producing bacteria. However, *Escherichia coli* and *Enterococci* do not usually produce urease. *Helicobacter pylori* is present in the upper gastrointestinal tracts of more than 50% of the population and while associated with peptic ulcer disease is of no recognised importance with respect to the urinary tract. *Ureaplasma urealyticum* is a mycoplasma bacterium of low pathogenicity that comprises part of the normal genital flora of many men and women. Gram-positive *Staphylococcus aureus* and *Staphylococcus epidermidis* can produce urease.

Urease catalyses the conversion of urea to ammonia which is subsequently hydrolysed to ammonium ions and hydroxyl ions:

$$H_2NCONH_2 + H_2O \rightarrow 2NH_3 + CO_2$$

$$2NH_3 + H_2O \rightarrow 2NH_4^+ + 2OH^- \left(\text{increase pH} > 7.2 \right)$$

It is hydroxyl (OH-) ions that are responsible for the alkalinisation of urine which is of fundamental significance to the pathophysiology of struvite stone formation. The presence of ammonia in alkaline urine (pH > 7.2) leads to the precipitation of magnesium ammonium phosphate (struvite) crystals which can lead to staghorn stone formation. Specific therapeutic measures for struvite stones therefore include urinary acidification, use of short-term and long-term antibiotics, and the use of urease inhibitors such as acetohydroxamic acid. Percutaneous chemolysis may be combined with ESWL for selective patients with staghorn stones who are not fit for percutaneous nephrolithotomy (Figure 16.2).

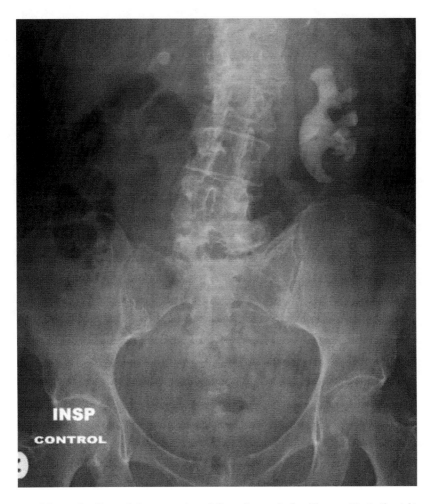

Figure 16.2   Plain abdominal radiograph demonstrating a left staghorn calculus. The opacities in the right upper quadrant are gallstones.

Q4. Answer B

The success of ESWL depends on factors that relate to the stone characteristics, the renal anatomy, the patient anatomy and the type of lithotriptor. Stone factors include the stone size, hardness, and location within the kidney. Success rates for lower pole stones are less than for stones located in the renal pelvis or other calyces. For example, in the Lower Pole I study only 21% of patients with stones larger than 10 mm located in a lower pole calyx were stone free after lithotripsy [5]. Adverse anatomic features include an infundibulopelvic angle <90 degrees and a narrow (<5 mm) or long (>30 mm) calyceal infundibulum [6]. The role for adjunctive measures to improve the outcome of ESWL for lower pole stones such as PDI (percussion, diuresis and inversion) is yet to be established.

The effectiveness of lithotripsy is also dependent on the hardness of the stone. For example, calcium oxalate monohydrate, dicalcium phosphate dihydrate (brushite) and cystine stones are relatively resistant to shockwaves although they are not contraindications to ESWL. Uric acid stones are radiolucent and must therefore be localised using ultrasound rather than fluoroscopy but are soft and may fragment well with lithotripsy.

Obesity reduces the effectiveness of ESWL and skin to stone difference has been shown to be an independent predictor of success [7]. Modern lithotriptors are less effective than the Dornier HM3 lithotriptor but are safer, better tolerated and do not require general anaesthesia. A recent meta-analysis has shown that reducing the shockwave frequency from 120 to 60–90 per minute improves stone clearance [8].

Q5. Answer C

All stone formers independent of their risk of developing further stones should follow general preventative measures to modify their risk. Patients should be encouraged to maintain a fluid intake of 2.5–3.0 L/day which should be increased as necessary to ensure a diuresis of 2.0–2.5 L/day. Most fluids can be consumed although some carbonated drinks, such as cola, contain phosphoric acid which may increase the risk of stone formation. Lemon juice increases urinary citrate and so reduces the risk of calcium oxalate stones. Although orange juice also increases urinary citrate, it raises oxalate levels and so is not recommended.

Patients should be advised to eat a healthy and balanced diet. However, foods rich in oxalate (for example, chocolate, nuts, rhubarb, tea) should be limited or avoided particularly in those patients with hyperoxaluria. Excessive dietary animal protein may cause hypocitraturia, hyperuricosuria, hyperoxaluria and acidic urine thereby encouraging stone formation. High salt intake increases the risk of urolithiasis by causing increased tubular calcium excretion and hypocitraturia. Therefore, not more than 3–5 g sodium should be consumed per day.

Patients often ask about dietary calcium and whether hard water (containing a high mineral content typically including calcium carbonate) in their locality caused their kidney stone. The data regarding water hardness are controversial but suggest that any increased lithogenic salt excretion may be neutralised by a greater excretion of stone inhibitors such as citrate and magnesium. On the other hand, there is good evidence that restricting dietary calcium actually increases the risk of stone formation through the reciprocal absorption of oxalate in the gut. A randomised study that compared the 5-year risk of stone recurrence in patients with a normal calcium, low salt and low protein diet to a low-calcium diet found a relative risk of

0.49 (95% CI 0.24-0.98, p-0.04) [9]. At least 1000 mg calcium should be consumed each day although calcium supplementation is generally not recommended except in some cases of enteric hyperoxaluria.

Calcium oxalate stones can be predominately calcium oxalate monohydrate or calcium oxalate dihydrate. Patients who have calcium oxalate monohydrate stones are often found to have hyperoxaluria in their metabolic workup, whereas those with calcium oxalate dehydrate stones are more likely to have hypercalciuria.

Q6. Answer D

ESWL relies on shockwave generation, a shockwave focussing, a coupling mechanism and a means of radiological imaging to localise the stone. Shockwaves may be generated at focal point F1 using electrohydraulic, piezoelectrical or electromagnetic lithotriptors. They are focussed, often by an ellipsoid dish, and converge on focal point F2, where stone fragmentation occurs.

Anticoagulation with warfarin is an absolute contraindication to ESWL and aspirin therapy should be withheld. Pregnancy, evidence of urinary sepsis and the presence of a calcified arterial aneurysm in the vicinity of the stone are also contraindications to ESWL.

Stone hardness is an important factor in predicting the likelihood of success of ESWL and can be estimated according to Hounsfield Units on non-contrast CT [10]. Stones with density >1,000 HU are less likely to fragment and it may be worth considering alternative treatment modalities in these cases. Cystine stones either respond well to ESWL or poorly which may reflect different stereoscopic crystalline structures.

According to a recent EAU/AUA meta-analysis, stone-free rates were significantly better for distal ureteric stones <10 mm and >10 mm and for proximal ureteric stones >10 mm treated with ureteroscopy (URS) compared to ESWL. Stone-free rates for mid-ureteric stones treated by URS and ESWL did not differ significantly [11].

A meta-analysis has shown that a shockwave rate of 1 Hz is optimal for stone fragmentation [8]. Data regarding the risk of developing hypertension and diabetes are controversial and insufficient to allow specific recommendations.

Q7. Answer D

Horseshoe kidneys represent a common congenital renal anomaly with an incidence of 1:400. They are twice as common in men and are associated with certain genetic conditions such as Turner's syndrome. Persistence of an isthmus, typically between the lower renal poles, arrests renal ascent usually at the level of the inferior mesenteric artery. As the kidney ascends, it takes a highly variable arterial blood supply from the aorta, iliac vessels and inferior mesenteric artery and this predisposes to a greater risk of bleeding with PCNL. An arteriogram should be considered prior to undertaking open surgery on a horseshoe kidney. There is also a failure of medial rotation of the kidneys that results in a medial orientation of the renal calyces and the isthmus causes the lower pole calyces to be deviated inwards.

ESWL is not contraindicated although the passage of stone fragments may be restricted by concomitant PUJ obstruction that is often seen in horseshoe kidneys as a result of high and medial insertion of the ureter into the renal pelvis. URS and PCNL are also treatment options for stones in horseshoe kidneys. The medially placed calyces should be considered when obtaining access for PCNL, and the incidence of colonic injury may be higher (Figure 16.3).

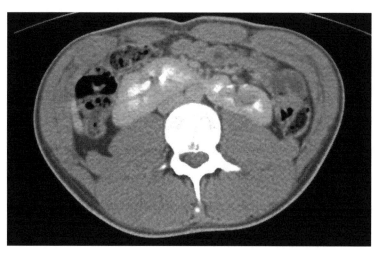

Figure 16.3 Axial computerised tomogram showing a horseshoe kidney. Note the position of the colon with respect to percutaneous renal access.

Q8. Answer A

Cystinuria like most inborn errors of metabolism is inherited in an autosomal recessive pattern with the gene defect located on Chromosome 2. It has been classified into three types (I, II and III) according to the specific gene mutation although this differentiation is of little clinical relevance. The incidence of heterozygous cystinuria is about 1 in 20,000 and these individuals are at high risk of recurrent cystine urolithiasis. Patients with cystinuria have defective absorption in the jejunum of cystine, and the other dibasic amino acids ornithine, lysine and arginine. The reabsorption of these amino acids in the proximal convoluted tubule of the kidney is also abnormal leading to high levels in the urine. Cystine, in contrast to ornithine, lysine and arginine, is relatively insoluble at physiological urine pH and has a pKa of 8.3. At pH < 7.0 the solubility of cystine is approximately 250 mg/L but at pH > 7.5 its solubility increases considerably to more than 500 mg/L [12]. Patients with heterozygous cystinuria excrete <200 mg/day and usually do not form stones whereas cystine excretion in homozygous cystinurics is typically 600–1400 mg/day.

Cystinurics usually present with their first stone episode in the second or third decade of life and represent a particularly challenging group of patients to treat. Cystine stones may be managed surgically by ESWL, URS, PCNL although ESWL may be less effective because they are hard. Also, cystine stones are poorly radio-opaque as they do not contain calcium and are visible only because of the disulphide bonds between the *cysteine* molecules.

Prevention of stone formation is the primary objective and patients should be advised to maintain a fluid intake of 2.5–3.0 L/day. They should also be referred to a dietician who will recommend a low methionine diet. Methionine, which is metabolised to cystine, is found in high concentrations in animal protein which should therefore be restricted. Patients are advised to alkalinise their urine with potassium citrate solution (10 mL tds) aiming for pH 7.0–8.0. However, potassium citrate solution is unpalatable and often poorly tolerated. An alternative, although not readily available in the UK, is potassium citrate tablets.

When these measures fail to adequately prevent stone formation, drugs which bind to cystine and thereby increase its solubility may be considered. D-Penicillamine binds cystine but is associated with considerable side effects such as skin rash, oral ulceration and gastrointestinal upset and has largely been superseded by tiopronin (Thiola) 1000 mg/day in divided doses. Vitamin C may increase the solubility of cystine but in high doses can cause hyperoxaluria that may predispose to stones of other types.

Q9. Answer C

The incidence of bladder calculi in the Western world has been declining because of improved nutrition and better control of urinary tract infection. However, in the developing world, bladder stones remain a significant problem especially in the paediatric population because of malnutrition and low phosphate diets.

Certain conditions predispose to bladder calculi formation in the adult population. Bladder outflow obstruction leading to incomplete bladder emptying and urinary stasis is a common cause of bladder stones and was once considered an absolute indication for bladder outflow surgery. However, a recent study that evaluated men with bladder calculi using pressure-flow studies found that only about half had bladder outflow obstruction [13]. Moreover, these findings were maintained even after stone surgery suggesting that the presence of the stone within the bladder did not affect the urodynamics results. Patients with long-term indwelling catheters, spinal cord injury patients and those with enteric bladder augmentations are also at higher risk of bladder calculi.

Open cystotomy is still considered by many urologists to be an excellent operation for large (>3 cm) bladder stones and may be combined with an open prostatectomy. However, the holmium laser now allows fragmentation of even very large bladder calculi and where bladder outflow surgery is also required it can be used to resect or enucleate the prostate [14].

Q10. Answer D

Analgesia should be offered as a priority to patients presenting with severe pain consistent with a diagnosis of acute ureteric colic.

NSAIDs should be considered initially as they provide effective relief from the pain of ureteric colic. NSAIDs inhibit cyclo-oxygenase and thereby inhibit prostaglandin synthesis from arachidonic acid. Prostaglandins mediate inflammation as well as pain through the sensitisation of nerve endings. Prostaglandins also act on afferent arterioles in the kidney causing vasodilatation. Inhibition of prostaglandin synthesis by NSAIDs therefore causes afferent arteriolar vasoconstriction which reduces renal blood flow, glomerular filtration rate and intrarenal pressure. Therefore, it may relieve the pain caused by distension of the collecting system associated with ureteric obstruction.

A Cochrane review and meta-analysis demonstrated lower pain scores with NSAIDs in 10 of 13 studies that compared NSAIDs with opioids for acute ureteric colic. Furthermore, patients treated with NSAIDs required less 'rescue' medication (need for further analgesia within 4 hours of administration) than those treated with opioids. Most studies showed a lower incidence of adverse effects with NSAIDs and vomiting was significantly less than in patients treated with opioids (RR 0.35, p < 0.00001) [15]. Pethidine particularly was associated with a higher rate of vomiting and should therefore be avoided in instances where an opioid is to be used. A further Cochrane review in 2015 was unable to determine which NSAID was the most effective [16].

Q11. Answer D

Most distal ureteric stones can be accessed with a rigid ureteroscope where surgical treatment is indicated. Flexible ureteroscopes facilitate the treatment of stones in the proximal ureter and pelvicalyceal system of the kidney. On the other hand, for distal ureteric stones flexible ureteroscopes are unwieldy and may easily slip out of the ureteric orifice.

Technological advances over recent years have led to the development of increasingly thin ureteroscopes that also provide exceptionally high resolution images. For example, the Stortz

Flex-X® shaft is 8.5 F which tapers to 7.5 F at the tip. A single lever control allows 270° active deflection of the tip in both upwards and downwards directions. The Olympus URF-P5® has a very slender tip that measures only 5.3 F. It has a maximal upward deflection of 180° and downward deflection of 275° to aid access to the lower pole. The working channels for most flexible ureteroscopes are 3.6 F.

The new digital flexible ureteroscope incorporates a distal video sensor and LEDs for illumination and therefore do not rely on fibre optics for light and image transmission. This results in better image quality although the shaft size and tip size are relatively larger. Furthermore, because of this digital ureteroscopes have limited manoeuvrability of the distal tip compared to fibre-optic flexible ureteroscopes.

Single-use flexible ureteroscopes have been on the market since 2015, and are made by a number of companies. There are digital single-use ureteroscopes available.

Q12. Answer E

A patient with a large stone in the renal pelvis should be fully counselled regarding the treatments that are available to them. A surveillance approach is seldom appropriate for a stone of this size given the high risk of potential complications. For patients with asymptomatic renal stones smaller than 1.5 cm, observation may be appropriate if they are fully informed of the risk of experiencing a symptomatic episode and the potential need for intervention. For example, in a cohort study that included 107 patients, the cumulative 5-year incidence of a symptomatic episode was 48.5% [17]. On the other hand, a prospective randomised controlled trial that compared surveillance with ESWL for small asymptomatic calyceal stones found no significant differences in stone-free rate, quality of life, renal function, symptoms or hospital admissions. However, surveillance was associated with a greater risk of needing more invasive treatment [18].

For a stone of this size (1.5 cm) located in the renal pelvis or upper or mid-zone calyces, ESWL may be effective but the patient should be advised that more than one treatment may be required. ESWL should not be considered first-line treatment for stones larger than 1.5 cm situated in lower pole calyces because of unfavourable outcomes. Similarly, stone size is inversely proportional to the effectiveness of flexible ureteroscopy and patients with large renal stones should be warned of the potential need for a staged procedure.

PCNL should be considered for stones larger than 2 cm because of reduced effectiveness of ESWL, the potential need for multiple treatments and the increased risk of complications such as colic and steinstrasse. PCNL may also be appropriate for a 1.5-cm stone in the renal pelvis for a patient who desires a single treatment and accepts the greater risk of significant morbidity compared to ESWL or URS. Laparoscopic or open endopyelotomy is not recommended for stones smaller than 2 cm and is generally reserved for special cases such as large stone burdens, previous failed PCNL, obesity or renal anatomical abnormalities.

Q13. Answer D

Ureteric stents may be used to relieve ureteric obstruction or be inserted prophylactically where obstruction is anticipated; for example, prior to ESWL for large (>2 cm) renal stones or after ureteroscopy. Indications for stenting following ureteroscopy may be remembered using the acronym SPOILED (Solitary kidney, Perforated ureter, Obstructed kidney/Oedema, Infection, Large residual stone burden, Elective second procedure anticipated, Dilatation of ureteric orifice to more than 10 F).

Pyonephrosis may be relieved with either a ureteric stent or percutaneous nephrostomy (PCN). One of the advantages of PCN is that it may be inserted under local anaesthesia thereby obviating the need for general anaesthesia in a patient who may be unstable due to sepsis or hyperkalaemia. That said, some clinicians will place stents without a GA, especially in women. Furthermore, a PCN may require less instrumentation of the urinary tract and reduce the risk of exacerbating sepsis. On the other hand, PCN requires the skills of an experienced interventional radiologist and where this expertise is not available a retrograde stent inserted by an experienced urologist may be a better option. The literature to date supports both methods of decompression [19,20].

Pearle randomised 42 patients with obstructing ureteric calculi to either PCN or retrograde ureteric stent [19]. There were no significant differences in time to resolution of fever or white cell count. There was one failed PCN which was salvaged with a retrograde stent. Length of stay was longer for PCN but ureteric stent was twice as expensive. In another randomised controlled trial Mokhmalji found that PCN was superior to retrograde ureteric stent insertion [20]. Failure rate was lower (0% vs. 20%), need for prolonged antibiotic therapy was reduced and PCN dwell time was less than for retrograde stents.

Ureteric stents may encrust rapidly in susceptible individuals but some may be left in-situ for one year; for example, the Percuflex® stent.

A systematic review and meta-analysis of five randomised placebo-controlled trials that included 461 patients suggested that administration of alpha-blockers reduced urinary symptom and body pain scores in patients with ureteric stents [21].

Q14. Answer C

Hyperoxaluria may be classified as primary, enteric or idiopathic. Primary hyperoxaluria (Types I and II) is inherited as an autosomal recessive condition that causes defective metabolism of glyoxalate in the liver and excess levels of endogenous oxalate. Enteric hyperoxaluria may occur in patients with functionally or anatomically abnormal small bowel. Oxalate normally complexes with calcium to form an insoluble salt that is excreted in the faeces. However, in conditions such as inflammatory bowel disease or after small bowel resection, the malabsorption of fatty acids leads to the saponification of calcium resulting in increased oxalate absorption from the colon. Similarly, a low-calcium diet encourages the absorption of oxalate from the bowel and should not be recommended to patients who form calcium oxalate stones [9].

Ethylene glycol (anti-freeze) induces hyperoxaluria and is commonly used in experimental animal studies to investigate calcium oxalate urolithiasis. Ascorbic acid (vitamin C) is converted to oxalate in the liver and may cause hyperoxaluria.

Oxalobacter formigenes is an anaerobic bacterium which colonises the large intestine of humans and causes the degradation of oxalate. It is important in the metabolism of calcium oxalate and its absence in the intestine following treatment with broad spectrum antibiotics such as quinolones may increase the risk of calcium stone formation.

Q15. Answer B

The HM1 (Human Machine 1) lithotriptor was developed in 1980 by the German aerospace company Dornier following research into the effects of shock waves on metal parts of supersonic aircraft. Four years later, the HM3 lithotriptor was introduced into clinical practice and remains amongst the most effective devices to fragment renal calculi. Its main drawback is that it requires general anaesthesia and immersion of the patient in a water bath. The shock waves are generated when a high-voltage electrical current passes across an underwater spark-gap electrode, creating a vaporisation bubble, which then rapidly collapses. The shock waves are focussed by an elliptical dish, angulated to avoid interference of the bubbles with transmission of the shock wave energy through the water to the patient.

Second-generation lithotriptors commonly use piezoelectric or electromagnetic generators as the energy source. These devices are more portable that the electrohydraulic lithotriptors such as the HM3 machine. In electromagnetic lithotriptors, such as the Stortz Modulith®, electrical energy applied to a magnetic coil results in the generation of a shock wave. Shock waves are focussed to a small focal zone (F2), which has the advantage of minimising collateral damage but may compromise fragmentation rates as the kidney and stone move with respiration. Shock wave generation in piezoelectric lithotriptors, for example the Wolf Piezolith 3000®, is achieved through the application of electricity to multiple ceramic crystals arranged around a hemispherical dish.

Q16. Answer D

Renal tubular acidosis (RTA) is a family of diseases characterised by failure of tubular H^+ secretion and urinary acidification. Type 1 RTA is the failure of H^+ secretion in the distal nephron tubules and is characterised by hyperchloraemic metabolic acidosis (normal anion gap), a high urinary pH (>5.5, alkaline urine) and low serum bicarbonate. The disease also has low sodium levels, there is a female predominance and due to the low citrate they are predisposed to calcium stones and in particular calcium phosphate stones. The condition is treated with potassium citrate solution. In Type 2 RTA, there is a failure of bicarbonate reabsorption (loss) in the proximal tubule of the nephron with similar characteristics to Type 1 RTA except citrate levels are normal therefore no stones form. The ammonium chloride acidification test (100 mg/kg) is one of the tests used to diagnose RTA with a urinary pH of >5.5 indicative of a failure of urinary acidification, and supportive of the diagnosis of dRTA.

Treatment of distal RTA include correction of the metabolic acidosis, with potassium citrate being one of the treatment options.

Q17. Answer C

Hypercalciuria is defined as >4 mg/kg/24 hours or >7 mmol (men) or >6 mmol (women). Hypercalciuria can classified into idiopathic (50%), absorptive (from gut), renal leak or resorptive (from bone). In absorptive hypercalciuria, excessive calcium is absorbed from the gut leading to increased renal filtration and reduced renal reabsorption due to low parathyroid hormone and associated raised urinary phosphate (fasting urinary calcium is normal). Impaired tubular reabsorption of calcium (renal leak) occurs in 5%–10% of calcium stone formers and is characterised by fasting hypercalciuria with secondary hyperparathyroidism (raised PTH) but without hypercalcaemia. Resorptive hypercalciuria is almost always due to primary hyperparathyroidism which accounts for 3%–5% of all cases of hypercalciuria. The increased PTH levels leads to release of calcium from the bones as well as increasing calcium and vitamin D absorption from the bone and reducing calcium renal excretion from the distal tubule resulting in hypercalciuria (Table 16.1). Excess salt intake can result in hypercalciuria, as sodium and calcium are co-transported in the kidney. Hypercalciuria is most commonly associated with calcium oxalate dihydrate stones.

Table 16.1 Summary of the discriminating features of the different causes of hypercalciuria

	Absorptive	**Renal**	**Resorptive**
Serum calcium	Normal	Normal	Elevated
Parathyroid hormone levels	Low	Elevated (secondarily)	Elevated (primarily)
Fasting urinary calcium	Normal	Elevated	Elevated
Intestinal calcium absorption	Elevated (primarily)	Elevated (secondarily)	Elevated (secondarily)

Q18. Answer A

The most important factor in uric acid stone formation is low urinary pH as most patients have normal urinary uric acid levels. Uric acid solubility is significantly reduced when urinary pH is <5.5. Other important factors include low urine volume and a hyperuricosuria. Low urinary volume can more commonly occur in patients with chronic diarrhoeal conditions, ileostomies, excessive sweating or poor oral intake. Hyperuricosuria occurs in addition to hyperuricaemia in patients with primary gout, myeloproliferative conditions and Lesch-Nyhan syndrome. Hyperuricosuria occurs in patients without raised serum urate levels due to some medications (thiazides or salicylates) and excessive intake of dietary meats.

Q19. Answer E

Penicillin, cephalosporin and macrolide antibiotics are considered safe to use in pregnancy. Nitrofurantoin is also safe for most of pregnancy but should be avoided towards term due to an increased risk of neonatal haemolysis. Trimethoprim is a folate antagonist and should be avoided, especially in the first trimester during organogenesis. There is a risk of auditory or vestibular nerve damage with gentamicin and therefore should not be used in pregnancy. There is limited information on tazocin or carbapenems with manufactures advising to use only if the potential benefit outweighs the risk in more severe infections.

Q20. Answer A

The most common types of urinary stones are composed of calcium oxalate (60%–70%) followed by calcium phosphate (10%–20%), infection stones (10%–15%) and then uric acid stones (5%–10%). Cystine stones occur in <1% of cases.

EMQs – ANSWERS

Q21. Answer B

Q22. Answer A

Q23. Answer K

Q24. Answer C

Q25. Answer A

Q26. Answer C

Q27. Answer E

The likelihood of spontaneous passage of ureteric stones is related to stone size and position. The evidence regarding spontaneous stone passage (SSP) of ureteric stones according to stone size is based historically on the 2007 joint EAU/AUA Guideline for the Management of Ureteral Calculi. This meta-analysis reported a spontaneous stone passage rate of 68% for stones smaller than 5 mm compared to 47% for stones larger than 5 mm [11]. It is intuitive that distal ureteric stones are more likely to pass than more proximal stones. A study of 378 patients with ureteric stones found that 22% of proximal, 46% of mid- and 71% of distal stones passed spontaneously [22]. Stone size has also been shown to affect the time taken for the stone to pass [23]. A period of observation is therefore recommended by the 2019 EAU guidelines panel in patients with small stones (<6 mm) who are fully informed and have no evidence of complications such as infection, deteriorating renal failure or uncontrolled pain [24]. It is a particularly good option in pregnancy where spontaneous stone passage rates are high [1].

The role of medical expulsive therapy (MET) in the spontaneous passage of ureteric calculi has recently been called into question by new high quality data from three well-designed, multicentre, placebo-controlled, double-blinded randomised controlled trials (RCT) which have shown limited or no benefit using alpha-blockers [25–27]. Hollingsworth et al. [28] subsequently published a meta-analysis of 55 trials which including the new studies above and concluded that MET promotes stone passage of large stones located in any part of the ureter. Opponents of this analysis contest their findings as the majority of studies included were small and from single centres with poor methodological quality which therefore limits the strength of their conclusions. Although the majority of UK urologists have now moved away from using MET in their practice, the EAU 2019 guideline panel have concluded that MET seems to be efficacious in patient with ureteric stones with the greatest benefit in larger and more distal stones [24]. If considering to offer MET patients should be informed that the evidence is controversial, its use is 'off label' and be made aware of the potential side effects (low blood pressure, retrograde ejaculation and stuffy nose).

Extracorporeal shockwave lithotripsy is recommended as treatment for stones up to 2 cm in all positions within the kidney other than in the lower pole [24]. A meta-analysis undertaken on behalf of the EAU and AUA in 2007 suggested that for proximal ureteric stones smaller than 1 cm, ESWL is more effective than ureteroscopic treatment [11]. However, for proximal ureteric stones larger than 1 cm clearance rates appeared better for ureteroscopy than lithotripsy. This may be explained in that the effectiveness of lithotripsy is dependent on stone size, whereas the effectiveness of ureteroscopic stone management is less influenced by stone size [11].

Where function is well preserved in a kidney containing a staghorn calculus, the stone should be removed by percutaneous nephrolithotomy. Where the kidney is non-functioning or poorly functioning (<15%), the patient should be counselled regarding simple nephrectomy.

Q28. Answer B

Q29. Answer H

Q30. Answer A

Q31. Answer F

Q32. Answer G

All stone patients should be advised to maintain a good fluid intake of 2.5–3.0 L/day; research has shown a significant reduction in risk of stone recurrence in those maintaining a high intake of water [29]. Attempts should be made to maintain a diuresis of 2.0–2.5 L accounting for environmental variations.

Urinary alkalinisation is important in the management of patients with both cystine stones and uric acid calculi. Sodium bicarbonate and potassium citrate are commonly used agents. Sodium bicarbonate is taken by mouth (325 to 2000 mg orally 1 to 4 times a day) and the dose titrated according to response. Common side effects include bloating and flatulence, but it may lead to salt and water retention and can worsen hypertension. The high sodium intake can lead to increased calcium absorption from the bowel and may increase the risk of calcium oxalate stones. Potassium citrate solution (10–20 mL three times per day) is again titrated according to urinary pH. It has a foul taste and compliance is less than 50%. Potassium citrate tablets are an alternative but are not available in the United Kingdom. Sodium citrate may also be used as a more palatable alternative. The target pH reflects the pKa of the stone constituents (for example, cystine – pKa 8.3, urate – pKa 5.8).

Hyperuricosuric patients are at risk of calcium oxalate stones [30]. They should be advised to modify their purine intake by reducing their consumption of animal protein. Urinary alkalinisation should be combined with allopurinol if dietary modification fails to prevent hyperuricosuria. Patients with uric acid stones and hyperuricosuria with or without hyperuricaemia should be given allopurinol (100–300 mg/day)

Thiazide diuretics such as bendroflumethiazide or chlorthalidone increase calcium reabsorption in the proximal and distal tubules. They should be considered in patients with idiopathic or absorptive hypercalciuruia. Side effects include impaired glucose tolerance, gout and erectile dysfunction. Hypokalaemia may require potassium supplementation. The benefits of treatment of absorptive hypercalciuria with thiazides may not be sustained after the initial few years of therapy [31].

Q33. Answer A

Q34. Answer A

Q35. Answer B

Q36. Answer F

Q37. Answer C

Q38. Answer E

All first-time stone formers should have their serum calcium, urate and creatinine checked. Hypercalcaemia demands an evaluation of parathyroid hormone levels to look for primary hyperparathyroidism, which is usually treated surgically. A recent study has suggested a four-fold increased prevalence of stones in patients with hyperparathyroidism compared to the general population [32].

Renal tubular acidosis (RTA) comprises a collection of disorders that result in a hyperchloraemic metabolic acidosis. It may be classified clinically into four types:

Type 1 – Distal RTA – 'complete' (low bicarbonate on blood gas analysis) or 'incomplete' (normal bicarbonate on blood gas analysis)

- Failure to excrete acid (protons) in the distal nephron.
- Hypokalaemia is common.
- Urine pH > 5.4 on ammonium chloride loading test.
- Calcium phosphate stone formation due to hypocitraturia, hypercalciuria and increased urine pH.
- A cause of nephrocalcinosis (calcium deposition within the renal parenchyma).

Type 2 – Proximal RTA

- Rare
- Associated with Fanconi syndrome
- Defect in the reabsorption of bicarbonate in the proximal tubule
- Urinary acidification maintained as distal acid excretion is normal
- Stones uncommon

Type 3 – A mixture of Types 1 and 2, which affects infants

Type 4 – Hypoaldosteronism

- Common in diabetic nephropathy and interstitial renal disease

Gout arises secondary to hyperuricaemia, which may result from a number of causes such as diet, genetic predisposition or underexcretion of uric acid. Ninety percent of patients with gout have a build up of uric acid as a result of inability to excrete sufficient amounts of urate in the urine. A small proportion of patients have hyperuricaemia as a result of overproduction such as in cases of Lesch-Nyhan syndrome. The prevalence of urolithiasis in patients with gout (10%–20%) is approximately twice as high as the general population [33]. Patients with hyperuricos-uria are also at an increased risk of calcium oxalate stones.

Q39. Answer A

Q40. Answer C

Q41. Answer B

Q42. Answer D

Q43. Answer E

The tipless nitinol stone retrieval basket has a 1.9 Fr sheath and may be passed through flex-ible ureteroscopes with minimal effect on scope deflection. It is well suited to remove renal stone fragments and the tipless design reduces the risk of urothelial trauma and thus minimises bleeding. Tipless baskets may also be used to reposition lower pole stones into upper pole caly-ces for more effective laser fragmentation.

Whenever a basket is used to retrieve ureteric stones or fragments, the surgeon has to consider the safety and effectiveness of the device. In an unstented ureter, extreme caution should be exercised. Under these circumstances tri-radiate graspers are often safer as they will release a stone which is too large to extract rather than damage or avulse the ureter. On the other hand, multiple small stone fragments in the distal part of a previously stented ureter may be more effectively removed with a basket.

Stone cone® and Entrap® are anti-retropulsion devices that may be used to secure a stone within the ureter while it is treated with the holmium laser and prevent it retrograde movement to the kidney. This is sensible if a flexible ureteroscope is not available.

Pedunculated ureteric polyps and papillary lesions suspicious for urothelial carcinoma may be effectively removed or biopsied using a flat wire basket. Often the volume of tissue retrieved is better than with ureteroscopic biopsy forceps. For flat urothelial lesions biopsy forceps are the most appropriate instrument.

Q44. Answer G

Q45. Answer D

Q46. Answer A

Q47. Answer G

Q48. Answer E

Q49. Answer E

Q50. Answer F

The holmium laser has a wavelength of 2132 nm, and its energy is readily absorbed by water, penetrating only 0.5 mm. It has found many uses in urology including lithotripsy, ablation of urothelial carcinomas and holmium laser enucleation of the prostate (HoLEP).

Both 200 and 365 μm fibres may be used with semi-rigid ureteroscopes to fragment ureteric calculi although the larger fibre occupies more working channel space, decreasing flow and also means that if there is a concurrent stone in the kidney for which flexible ureteroscopy is being attempted, a separate 200 micron fibre is likely to be required.

Fragmentation using the holmium laser is best undertaken with a higher energy, low frequency and short pulse width, while dusting is a lower energy, higher frequency and long pulse width. Cutting or ablation of tumour is most commonly undertaken using a setting of 1 J, 10 Hz and a long pulse width.

A 200 μm fibre is generally the better option for treatment of renal calculi with flexible ureteroscopy, particularly those in lower pole calyces.

HoLEP is undertaken with a 550-μm laser fibre, with the laser generator set at maximum power (100–120 W). Large bladder calculi that traditionally required open cystolithotomy can now be safely and effectively treated with the holmium laser, with a high energy and frequency.

Q51. Answer C

Q52. Answer E

Q53. Answer A

Q54. Answer B

Q55. Answer D

Q56. Answer D

Q57. Answer D

D-Penicillamine may be used to treat cystinuria. It binds to cystine forming a disulphide complex that is 50 times more soluble than cystine. Side effects are common affecting approximately 50% of patients. They include nausea, arthralgia, loss of taste and rash. Leukopaenia and thrombocytopaenia are also recognised side effects and bloods should therefore be checked every 1–2 weeks initially then every 4 weeks. Tiopronin (Thiola®) is a complexing thiol compound with similar side effects to penicillamine, although these occur much less commonly.

Captopril is a thiol ACE inhibitor that binds to cystine increasing its solubility 200 fold. ACE inhibitors may cause profound hypotension particularly after the first dose. They are contraindicated in patients with bilateral renal artery stenosis in whom they reduce glomerular filtration and result in progressive renal failure. They may cause rash, gastrointestinal disturbance and are associated with a persistent dry cough.

Potassium citrate solution is unpalatable and is associated with diarrhoea and nausea. These gastrointestinal symptoms may be reduced if the drug is taken with meals. Severe side effects include severe allergic reactions and those symptoms that may be attributable to hyperkalaemia such as muscle cramps and cardiac arrhythmias.

Q58. Answer E

Q59. Answer F

Q60. Answer E

Q61. Answer A

Most guidewires used in endourology are 150 cm in length. Their diameter is also indicated, typically ranging from 0.025 to 0.038 inches. They have either a stainless steel or a nitinol core and have a low-friction biocompatible coating. Nitinol (Nickel-Titanium/Naval Ordnance Laboratory) is a nickel-titanium alloy that is strong, flexible and when deformed and released resumes its original configuration. It is used as the core for some guidewires and in the manufacture of baskets and graspers in endourology. It is also used in the thermo-expandable Memokath® ureteric stents.

Guidewires may have either a straight tip or a 'J' tip, which may be particularly useful for impacted ureteric calculi. The Sensor® guidewire has a hydrophilic tip that may also help to negotiate difficult ureteric stones. Similarly the Terumo® guidewire has a hydrophilic coating throughout its length and should be wetted with saline or water before use, which renders it extremely 'slippery'. In general, nitinol-based wires and those that focus on lubricity are best suited for access, whereas wires with stiffer shafts are better for the passage of stents, sheaths and catheters.

The Amplatz Super Stiff® wire is a coiled stainless steel wire with a PTFE coating. It is often used for tract dilatation in percutaneous nephrolithotomy and may also be used to straighten dilated and tortuous ureters prior to retrograde ureteric stenting. The Bentson wire is a PTFE coated wire with a stainless steel core.

Q62. Answer A

Q63. Answer C

Q64. Answer D

Q65. Answer B

Q66. Answer B

Q67. Answer E

Q68. Answer B

Beta (β)-lactam antibiotics contain a β-lactam ring in their molecular structure, which act as an irreversible inhibitor of the enzyme transpeptidase, which is used by the bacteria to cross-link peptidoglycan in their cell walls. β-lactam antibiotics include penicillin derivatives (penams such as amoxicillin), cephalosporins (cephems such as cephalexin) and carbapenems (such as meropenem or itrapenem). Aminoglycosides (gentamicin) are important treatments against Gram-negative infections. They act by inhibiting protein synthesis by binding to ribosomal RNA, which disrupts the integrity of the bacterial cell wall membrane. Sulphonamides are one of the oldest groups of antibiotic compounds (trimethoprim-sulphonamide) in use. They are structurally similar to para-aminobenzoic acid (PABA) and act as a false substrate for the enzyme dihydrofolate synthase, which blocks the synthesis of folate. This results in inhibition of DNA synthesis and therefore bacterial cell growth. Fluoroquinolone (ciprofloxacin) antibiotics inhibit the enzyme DNA gyrase, which is essential for transcription bacterial DNA synthesis, and results in irreversible damage and bacterial cell death. Nitrofurantoin is reduced inside the bacterial cell by flavoproteins (nitrofuran reductase) to multiple intermediates that attack ribosomal proteins (ribosomal subunit 50 S and target 23 S ribosomal RNA, DNA and pyruvate metabolism (Table 16.2).

Table 16.2 Summary of common antibiotics mode of action and effect on bacteria

Antibiotic group	Mode of action	Effect on bacteria
Penicillin	Inhibition of cell wall synthesis	Bactericidal
Cephalosporins	Inhibition of cell wall synthesis	Bactericidal
Carbapenems	Inhibition of cell wall synthesis	Bactericidal
Fluoroquinolones	Inhibit DNA gyrase	Bactericidal
Trimethoprim	Inhibit folate synthesis	Bacteriostatic
Aminoglycosides	Inhibit ribosomal protein synthesis	Bactericidal
Nitrofurantoin	Inhibit ribosomal protein synthesis	Bactericidal

Q69. Answer C

Q70. Answer D

Q71. Answer E

Q72. Answer A

Q73. Answer F

Q74. Answer B

The urine sediment of stone formers can be examined using light microscopy for crystalluria. The common stone have unique crystals which can help in the identification of the common stone types (Table 16.3).

Table 16.3 Summary of the crystal shape of common stone using light microscopy of urinary sediment

Stone type	Crystal shape under light microscopy
Calcium oxalate monohydrate	Dumbbell
Calcium oxalate dihydrate	Envelope
Calcium phosphate	Flat shaped or wedge prisms
Struvite (magnesium ammonium phosphate)	Coffin-lid
Uric acid	Amorphous shard or plates
Cystine	Hexagonal

REFERENCES

1. Parulkar, B.G., et al., Renal colic during pregnancy: A case for conservative treatment. *J Urol*, 1998. **159**(2): 365–368.
2. Semins, M.J., B.J. Trock, and B.R. Matlaga, The safety of ureteroscopy during pregnancy: A systematic review and meta-analysis. *J Urol*, 2009. **181**(1): 139–143.
3. Ohmori, K., et al., Effects of shock waves on the mouse fetus. *J Urol*, 1994. **151**(1): 255–258.
4. Robertson, W.G., M. Peacock, and B.E. Nordin, Activity products in stone-forming and non-stone-forming urine. *Clin Sci*, 1968. **34**(3): 579–594.
5. Albala, D.M., et al., Lower pole I: A prospective randomized trial of extracorporeal shock wave lithotripsy and percutaneous nephrostolithotomy for lower pole nephrolithiasis-initial results. *J Urol*, 2001. **166**(6): 2072–2080.
6. Elbahnasy, A.M., et al., Lower-pole caliceal stone clearance after shockwave lithotripsy, percutaneous nephrolithotomy, and flexible ureteroscopy: Impact of radiographic spatial anatomy. *J Endourol*, 1998. **12**(2): 113–119.
7. Patel, T., et al., Skin to stone distance is an independent predictor of stone-free status following shockwave lithotripsy. *J Endourol*, 2009. **23**(9): 1383–1385.
8. Semins, M.J., B.J. Trock, and B.R. Matlaga, The effect of shock wave rate on the outcome of shock wave lithotripsy: A meta-analysis. *J Urol*, 2008. **179**(1): 194–197; discussion 197.
9. Borghi, L., et al., Comparison of two diets for the prevention of recurrent stones in idiopathic hypercalciuria. *N Engl J Med*, 2002. **346**(2): 77–84.
10. Pareek, G., N.A. Armenakas, and J.A. Fracchia, Hounsfield units on computerized tomography predict stone-free rates after extracorporeal shock wave lithotripsy. *J Urol*, 2003. **169**(5): 1679–1681.
11. Preminger, G.M., et al., 2007 Guideline for the management of ureteral calculi. *Eur Urol*, 2007. **52**(6): 1610–1631.
12. Mattoo, A. and D.S. Goldfarb, Cystinuria. *Semin Nephrol*, 2008. **28**(2): 181–191.
13. Millan-Rodriguez, F., et al., Treatment of bladder stones without associated prostate surgery: Results of a prospective study. *Urology*, 2005. **66**(3): 505–509.
14. D'Souza, N. and A. Verma, Holmium laser cystolithotripsy under local anaesthesia: Our experience. *Arab J Urol*, 2016. **14**(3): 203–206.
15. Holdgate, A. and T. Pollock, Nonsteroidal anti-inflammatory drugs (NSAIDs) versus opioids for acute renal colic. *Cochrane Database Syst Rev*, 2004. **2004**(1): Cd004137.
16. Afshar, K., et al., Nonsteroidal anti-inflammatory drugs (NSAIDs) and non-opioids for acute renal colic. *Cochrane Database of Syst Rev*, 2015. **2015**(6): CD006027.
17. Glowacki, L.S., et al., The natural history of asymptomatic urolithiasis. *J Urol*, 1992. **147**(2): 319–321.
18. Keeley, F.X., Jr., et al., Preliminary results of a randomized controlled trial of prophylactic shock wave lithotripsy for small asymptomatic renal calyceal stones. *BJU Int*, 2001. **87**(1): 1–8.
19. Pearle, M.S., et al., Optimal method of urgent decompression of the collecting system for obstruction and infection due to ureteral calculi. *J Urol*, 1998. **160**(4): 1260–1264.
20. Mokhmalji, H., et al., Percutaneous nephrostomy versus ureteral stents for diversion of hydronephrosis caused by stones: A prospective, randomized clinical trial. *J Urol*, 2001. **165**(4): 1088–1092.
21. Lamb, A.D., et al., Meta-analysis showing the beneficial effect of alpha-blockers on ureteric stent discomfort. *BJU Int*, 2011. **108**(11): 1894–1902.
22. Morse, R.M. and M.I. Resnick, Ureteral calculi: Natural history and treatment in an era of advanced technology. *J Urol*, 1991. **145**(2): 263–265.
23. Miller, O.F. and C.J. Kane, Time to stone passage for observed ureteral calculi: A guide for patient education. *J Urol*, 1999. **162**(3 Pt 1): 688–690; discussion 690-1.
24. European Association of Urology Guidelines on urolithiasis. 2019. http://uroweb.org/guideline/urolithiasis/
25. Pickard, R., et al., Medical expulsive therapy in adults with ureteric colic: a multicentre, randomised, placebo-controlled trial. *Lancet*, 2015. **386**(9991): 341–349.

26. Furyk, J.S., et al., Distal ureteric stones and tamsulosin: A double-blind, placebo-controlled, randomized, multicenter trial. *Ann Emerg Med*, 2016. **67**(1): 86–95.e2.
27. Sur, R.L., et al., Silodosin to facilitate passage of ureteral stones: A multi-institutional, randomized, double-blinded, placebo-controlled trial. *Eur Urol*, 2015. **67**(5): 959–964.
28. Hollingsworth, J.M., et al., Alpha blockers for treatment of ureteric stones: Systematic review and meta-analysis. *BMJ*, 2016. **355**: i6112.
29. Borghi, L., et al., Urinary volume, water and recurrences in idiopathic calcium nephrolithiasis: A 5-year randomized prospective study. *J Urol*, 1996. **155**(3): 839–843.
30. Coe, F.L. and A.G. Kavalach, Hypercalciuria and hyperuricosuria in patients with calcium nephrolithiasis. *N Engl J Med*, 1974. **291**(25): 1344–1350.
31. Preminger, G.M. and C.Y. Pak, Eventual attenuation of hypocalciuric response to hydrochlorothiazide in absorptive hypercalciuria. *J Urol*, 1987. **137**(6): 1104–1109.
32. Suh, J.M., J.J. Cronan, and J.M. Monchik, Primary hyperparathyroidism: Is there an increased prevalence of renal stone disease? *AJR Am J Roentgenol*, 2008. **191**(3): 908–911.
33. Kramer, H.J., et al., The association between gout and nephrolithiasis in men: The health professionals' follow-up study. *Kidney Int*, 2003. **64**(3): 1022–1026.

CHAPTER 17: URINARY TRACT INFECTIONS (UTI)

Nish Bedi, Ali Omar and Jas S. Kalsi

MCQs

Q1. Risk factors for UTI in postmenopausal women include all of the following, EXCEPT
   A. Atrophic vaginitis
   B. UTI before menopause
   C. Non-secretor status
   D. Smoking
   E. Cystocele

Q2. Screening for asymptomatic bacteriuria should NOT be performed in all of the following, EXCEPT
   A. Patients undergoing invasive genito-urinary surgery with risk of mucosal bleeding
   B. Patients with nephrostomy in-situ
   C. Postmenopausal women
   D. Women with diabetes
   E. Patients with spinal cord injury

Q3. Regarding the diagnosis of asymptomatic bacteriuria all the following are true, EXCEPT
   A. For women, a count of $\geq 10^5$ cfu/mL in voided volume in two consecutive samples is diagnostic.
   B. For men, a count of $\geq 10^5$ cfu/mL in voided volume in two consecutive samples is diagnostic.
   C. For patients with indwelling catheter, a count of $\geq 10^2$ cfu/mL in a single collected urine sample is diagnostic.
   D. For specimens collected with in and out catheter, a count of $\geq 10^3$ cfu/mL in collected urine is appropriate quantitative diagnostic criterion.
   E. For men with specimen collected using external condom catheter, $\geq 10^3$ cfu/mL is an appropriate quantitative diagnostic criterion.

Q4. Concerning UTI in pregnancy all the following are true, EXCEPT
   A. Asymptomatic bacteriuria detected should be eradicated with antibiotics.
   B. Women should not be screened for bacteriuria in the first trimester of pregnancy.
   C. Two consecutive specimens $> 10^5$ cfu/mL of the same bacteria is defined as significant bacteriuria.
   D. Avoid trimethoprim in the first trimester.
   E. Avoid sulfamethoxazole in the third trimester.

Q5. In patients with renal transplant all are true, EXCEPT
   A. Treat infection in recipient before transplant.
   B. Culture donor tissue samples and perfusate.
   C. Perioperative antibiotic prophylaxis should be given.
   D. Lifelong antibiotic prophylaxis should always be commenced after transplantation to prevent urinary infections.
   E. UTI is common after renal transplant.

Q6. For urinary catheters and UTI the following are false, EXCEPT
   A. 1%–2% of ambulatory patients develop UTI after single catheterisation.
   B. Open drainage indwelling catheter results in bacteriuria in 100% cases in 3–5 days.
   C. Biofilm develops in between catheter and the urethral mucosa.
   D. Up to 50% of patients catheterised for more than 28 days will suffer from catheter encrustation and blockade.
   E. Antibiotic prophylaxis decreases the rate of bacteriuria in patients on intermittent catheterisation.

Q7. Regarding UTI and immunoactive pro-
phylaxis all the following are true,
EXCEPT
   A. OM-89 can be recommended for female
      patients with recurrent UTI.
   B. Intravaginal probiotics restore vaginal
      lactobacilli.
   C. Probiotics containing *L. rhamnosus*
      GR-1 and *L. reuteri* RC-14 can prevent
      recurrent UTI.
   D. Proanthocyanidin is the active ingredient
      in probiotics.
   E. Probiotics prevent bacterial vaginosis.

Q8. The following factors suggest a compli-
cated UTI, EXCEPT
   A. Vesicoureteric reflux
   B. Radiation exposure to urothelium
   C. Bladder stone
   D. Older than 60 years
   E. Presence of nephrostomy

Q9. The following are true for *Escherichia coli*
(*E. coli*) uropathogenesis, EXCEPT
   A. Represents 80% of uncomplicated UTI.
   B. The virulence factors include adhesins
      and toxins.
   C. Non-urea-splitting pathogen.
   D. The endotoxins can precipitate systemic
      inflammatory response syndrome (SIRS).
   E. Endotoxins are recognised by receptors in
      cell cytoplasm.

Q10. Following are urea-splitting uropathogen,
EXCEPT
   A. *Proteus*
   B. *Klebsiella*
   C. *Pseudomonas*
   D. *Ureaplasma urealyticum*
   E. *Clostridium difficile*

Q11–16. Uropathogens
   A. *Clostridium difficile*
   B. Uropathogenic *Escherichia coli*
   C. Adhesins
   D. Endotoxins
   E. Urea-splitting bacteria
   F. P-fimbriae
   G. Type 1 pili
   H. >1.5

For the following statements below, choose the
most appropriate response from the list above.

Q11. Represents 80% of uncomplicated UTIs

Q12. FimH mannose binding pili

Q13. Structurally classified as
lipopolysaccharides

Q14. *Klebsiella*

Q15. Pyelonephritis

Q16. Invasion of bladder epithelium

Q17–21. Schistosomiasis
   A. A trematode
   B. Intestinal schistosomiasis
   C. Swim freely in fresh water
   D. Penetrates the human skin
   E. Primary sporocyst
   F. Miracidium

For each of the following aspects of schistosomiasis listed below, please choose the most appropriate description from the list above.

Q17. Cercariae

Q18. Miracidium

Q19. *Schistosoma mansoni*

Q20. *Schistosoma haematobium*

Q21. Released from eggs laid by adult
Schistosoma

Q22–26. Genito-urinary tuberculosis
   A. Acid fast bacilli
   B. Ethambutol
   C. Urine culture
   D. The doubling time for mycobacterium
      tuberculosis is
   E. Severe unilateral renal tuberculosis
      can cause
   F. Tuberculous epididymitis
   G. Rifampicin
   H. Xpert MTB/RIF assay (DNA-based PCR
      test)

For each of the following topics listed below,
please choose the most appropriate description
from the list above.

Q22. Ziehl–Neelsen stain

Q23. Optic neuritis

Q24. Lowenstein-Jensen culture medium

Q25. 15–20 hours

Q26. Hypertension

Q27–31. *Escherichia coli*
  A. Type 1 pili
  B. P-fimbriae
  C. 70%–95% cases
  D. Mannose resistant
  E. Proteinaceous component of the *E. coli* biofilm
  F. Cellulose

For each of the descriptions listed below, please choose the most appropriate answer from the list above.

Q27. Bladder epithelial invasion

Q28. Febrile non-obstructed pyelonephritis

Q29. *E. coli* the causative uropathogen in

Q30. Curli fimbriae

Q31. Afa/Dr adhesins

Q32–36. Antibiotics
  A. Binds to bacterial dihydrofolate reductase
  B. Inhibit bacterial DNA gyrase
  C. Inhibits cell wall biosynthesis
  D. Bind to 50S subunit of ribosomes
  E. Bind to 30S subunit of ribosomal RNA
  F. Mitochondrial DNA inactivation

For each of the antibiotics listed below, please choose the most appropriate mode of action from the list above.

Q32. Trimethoprim

Q33. Ciprofloxacin

Q34. Penicillins

Q35. Macrolides

Q36. Aminoglycosides

Q37–41. Uncomplicated UTI
  A. 70%–95% cases
  B. 5%–10% cases
  C. Suspected acute pyelonephritis
  D. Colony count of $\geq 10^3$ in symptomatic women.
  E. Is recommended
  F. Is not recommended

For each of the statements listed below, please choose the most appropriate answer from the list above.

Q37. *E. coli* are found to be causative pathogens.

Q38. *Staphylococcus saprophyticus* are causative pathogens.

Q39. Urine cultures are recommended.

Q40. The criteria for lab diagnosis of UTI.

Q41. Routine post-treatment urinalysis.

Q42–46. Prophylaxis against UTI
  A. Oral immunostimulant bacterial extract.
  B. Antibiotic cycling.
  C. *L. rhamnosus* GR-1.
  D. Proanthocyanidins A is the active ingredient.
  E. Local administration of estriol can reduce incidence of UTI.
  F. Routine *E. coli* vaccination.

For each of the descriptions listed below, please choose the most appropriate answer from the list above.

Q42. OM-89

Q43. Intravaginal probiotics

Q44. Cranberry

Q45. Postmenopausal women

Q46. Antimicrobial resistance can be prevented by

Q47–51. Pregnancy and UTI
  A. Third trimester and term
  B. Avoid in glucose 6 phosphate dehydrogenase deficiency
  C. First trimester of pregnancy
  D. Amoxicillin
  E. Trimethoprim
  F. Third trimester

For each of the descriptions listed below, please choose the most appropriate answer from the list above.

Q47. Contraindicated in first trimester.

Q48. Recommended in first trimester to treat asymptomatic bacteriuria.

Q49. Pregnant women should be screened for bacteria.

Q50. Nitrofurantoin.

Q51. Sulfamethoxazole should be avoided.

Q52–56. Epididymitis and orchitis
   A. Sexual partner should be treated.
   B. Gram staining of urethral smears.
   C. Urethra or the bladder.
   D. Unilateral.
   E. Develops in 20%–30% of post-pubertal men with mumps virus infection.
   F. Blood borne.
   G. Bilateral.
   H. Sexual contact.
   I. AFB smear and culture.

For each of the clinical descriptions listed below, please choose the most appropriate answer from the list above.

Q52. Mumps orchitis

Q53. Acute epididymitis is almost always

Q54. Typically, the organism reaches epididymis from

Q55. Microbiology of epididymitis can be determined through

Q56. In case of trachomatis epididymitis

Q57–61. Urological infections
   A. More common in diabetics.
   B. Von Hansemann cells are pathognomonic.
   C. Caseating granulomas.
   D. Falling CD4 count.
   E. Lipid-laden foamy macrophages.
   F. Mast cell infiltration of the lamina propria.

For each of the descriptions listed below, please choose the most appropriate answer from the list above.

Q57. Xanthogranulomatous pyelonephritis

Q58. Malakoplakia

Q59. Tuberculosis

Q60. HIV

Q61. Emphysematous pyelonephritis

MCQs – ANSWERS

Q1. Answer D

In older, often-institutionalised female patients, urinary tract catheterisation and functional status deterioration appear to be the most important risk factors associated with UTI. The other risk factors include non-secretor status of blood group antigens, UTIs before menopause, urinary incontinence, atrophic vaginitis, cystocele and large post-voiding residual urine.

Q2. Answer A

Screening for asymptomatic bacteriuria is not recommended for the following patients:

- Premenopausal, non-pregnant women
- Postmenopausal women
- Patients with well-controlled diabetes
- Residents of long-term care facilities
- Patients with an indwelling urethral catheter
- Patients with nephrostomy tubes or ureteric stent
- Patients with spinal cord injury
- Patients with candiduria
- Patients with renal transplants
- Patients with recurrent UTIs
- Patients with urinary tract reconstruction

Q3. Answer B

For asymptomatic bacteriuria in women a count of $\geq 10^5$ cfu/mL in voided volume in two consecutive samples is diagnostic, whereas only one sample is needed to be diagnostic for a man with no urinary symptoms In a single catheterised sample, a count may be as low as 10^2 cfu/mL to be diagnostic. The count can be slightly higher at 10^3 cfu/mL for an 'in and out' catheter or convene/condom catheter sample to be diagnostic.

Asymptomatic bacteriuria should only be treated in pregnant women or prior to transurethral surgery with a risk of mucosal bleeding.

Essential read: EAU guidelines on Urological Infections and NICE Quality Standards (QS90), List of Quality Statements (Urinary tract infections in adults)

Q4. Answer B

Pregnancy does not alter the diagnostic criteria; therefore, in an asymptomatic pregnant woman, bacteriuria is considered significant if two consecutive voided urine specimens grow $>10^5$ cfu/mL of the same bacterial species on quantitative culture; or a single catheterised specimen grows $>10^5$ cfu/mL of a uropathogen.

Pregnant women should be screened for bacteriuria during the first trimester. Asymptomatic bacteriuria detected in pregnancy should be eradicated with antimicrobial therapy, with a standard short course. Trimethoprim is a dihydrofolate reductase inhibitor preventing DNA replication. Sulfamethoxazole inhibits bacterial use of para-aminobenzoic acid (PABA) for synthesis of folic acid, needed in DNA synthesis.

Q5. Answer D

After the kidney is removed from its storage box, the effluent from the renal vein and surrounding fluid in the sterile plastic bags that contain the excised kidney should ideally be cultured because microorganisms are likely to have been introduced during the donation process.
Six months low-dose co-trimoxazole is recommended in renal transplant patients to prevent UTI.

Q6. Answer E

Catheters provide a surface for a bacterial biofilm formation and residual urine is increased through pooling below the catheter bulb. The biofilm forms on the surface of the catheter. The daily rate of colonisation is 5%, so that by 4 weeks almost 100% are colonised with bacteria. It is estimated that all long-term catheters are colonised with at least two organisms. In the UK, UTI is the most common hospital-acquired infection accounting for 23% of all infections and the majority of these are associated with catheters.

Q7. Answer D

OM-89 significantly reduced the incidence of UTI [1]. Intravaginal probiotics restore vaginal lactobacilli. Probiotics containing *L. rhamnosus* GR-1 and *L. reuteri* RC-14 can prevent recurrent UTI [2]. A type proanthocyanidins have been clinically demonstrated to attach to *E. coli* fimbriae, preventing the bacteria from attaching to the urinary tract or the urinary bladder [3]. Interesting read [4].

Q8. Answer D

A complicated UTI indicates there is an abnormality in the urinary tract, either innate or as a result of pathology or medical intervention.

Q9. Answer E

The spectrum of aetiological agents is similar in uncomplicated upper and lower UTIs, with *E. coli* the causative pathogen in 70%–95% of cases and *Staphylococcus saprophyticus* in 5%–10%. Occasionally, other Enterobacteriaceae, such as *Proteus mirabilis* and *Klebsiella* species are isolated [4,5]. Virulence factors prevent *E. coli* from immune recognition or even actively reduce an immune response. They include adhesins, toxins, iron acquisition systems and immune evasion mechanisms.

Pathogen recognition receptors Toll-like receptor (TLR) 4 and TLR5 appear the most important receptors for endotoxins, with TLR4 recognising lipopolysaccharide (LPS), as the major component of the cell wall in Gram-negative bacteria.

Q10. Answer E

Urea-splitting bacteria are *Proteus, Klebsiella, Pseudomonas, Providencia, Serratia* species, *Staphylococcus aureus* and *Ureaplasma urealyticum*. *Proteus mirabilis* accounts for more than half of all urease positive urinary infections [6]. Urea-splitting bacteria change the urine pH (>7.2) and allow easier precipitation of phosphate with several compounds, mainly ammonium and magnesium [7]. The result is struvite stones.

Q11. Answer B

Q12. Answer G

Q13. Answer D

Q14. Answer E

Q15. Answer F

Q16. Answer G

Most strains of uropathogenic *Escherichia coli* (UPEC) encode filamentous adhesive organelles called type 1 pili. Type 1 pilus adhesin, FimH, mediates not only bacterial adherence, but also invasion of human bladder epithelial cells [1]. In Gram-negative bacteria, specific lipopolysaccharides (LPS) represent some of the most toxic virulence factors of bacterial origin. LPS have no chemical homologs among human cells and are known as endotoxins [2]. *P-fimbriae* are involved in pyelonephritis [3].

Q17. Answer D

Q18. Answer C

Q19. Answer B

Q20. Answer A

Q21. Answer F

Infection with *Schistosoma* is known as schistosomiasis or bilharzia and is contracted from exposure to contaminated water. It is extremely important to remember the life cycle of *Schistosoma haematobium*, which is the species that affects the urinary tract. *Schistosoma mansoni* causes intestinal schistosomiasis. Miracidium is the larval stage after hatching from the egg, where the parasite swims to its first host usually a snail. Cercariae is the larval stage after leaving the snail which is able to penetrate human skin (Figure 17.1).

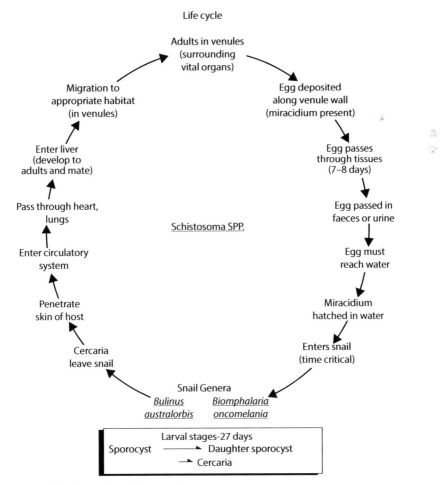

Figure 17.1   The life cycle in Schistosomiasis.

Q22. Answer A

Q23. Answer B

Q24. Answer C

Q25. Answer D

Q26. Answer E

Ziehl-Neelson stain is used to identify acid fast bacilli, most important of which is *Mycobacterium tuberculosis*. Ethambutol is contraindicated in optic neuritis. *Mycobacterium tuberculosis* is a slow-growing bacterium, with a doubling time of 15–20 hours, therefore culture and sensitivities can take 4–6 weeks. Unilateral renal tuberculosis has been associated with hypertension.

Q27. Answer A

Q28. Answer B

Q29. Answer C

Q30. Answer E

Q31. Answer D

Adhesion factors can be fimbrial or pili, which are polymeric hair-like structures or non-fimbrial which are shorter monomeric or trimeric structures. Type 1 pili (fimH mannose binding pili) has a critical role in initial attachment to uroepithelial cells resulting in epithelial invasion. It also binds N-linked oligomannose glycoproteins and uroplakin. Pyelonephritis-associated pili (P-fimbriae) is present in 80% of pyelonephritis isolates.

Afa/Dr adhesins bind the Dr (a+) blood group antigen present on the complement cascade regulator factor and have been shown to demonstrate mannose resistant strains.

Q32. Answer A

Q33. Answer B

Q34. Answer C

Q35. Answer D

Q36. Answer E

Quinolones rapidly inhibit DNA synthesis by promoting cleavage of bacterial DNA in the DNA-enzyme complexes of DNA gyrase and type IV topoisomerase, resulting in rapid bacterial death [4]. Penicillin kills susceptible bacteria by specifically inhibiting the transpeptidase that catalyses the final step in cell wall biosynthesis, the cross-linking of peptidoglycan [5]. Macrolides bind to 50S subunit of ribosomes (does not exist in human cells). More specifically to the peptidyl transferase site. The aminoglycosides primarily act by binding to the aminoacyl site of 16S ribosomal RNA within the 30S ribosomal subunit, leading to misreading of the genetic code and inhibition of translocation [6,7].

Q37. Answer A

Q38. Answer B

Q39. Answer C

Q40. Answer D

Q41. Answer F

Acute, uncomplicated UTIs in adults are seen mostly in women without any relevant structural and functional abnormalities within the urinary tract. *E. coli* is the commonest causative pathogen in 70%–95% of cases and *Staphylococcus saprophyticus* in 5%–10%. Occasionally, other Enterobacteriaceae, such as *Proteus mirabilis* and *Klebsiella* spp., are the isolated cause.

Urine dipstick testing, as opposed to urinary microscopy, is a reasonable alternative to urinalysis for the diagnosis of acute uncomplicated cystitis. Whereas urine cultures are recommended for those with suspected acute pyelonephritis, symptoms that do not resolve or recur within 2–4 weeks after the completion of treatment; and women who present with atypical symptoms.

A colony count of $>10^3$ cfu/mL of uropathogens is microbiologically diagnostic in women who present with symptoms of acute uncomplicated cystitis. The routine post-treatment urinalysis or urine cultures in asymptomatic patients are not indicated or recommended.

Q42. Answer A

Q43. Answer C

Q44. Answer D

Q45. Answer E

Q46. Answer B

OM-89 (Uro-Vaxomâ) has been shown to be more effective than placebo in several randomised trials and is therefore recommended for immunoprophylaxis in female patients with recurrent uncomplicated UTI. Intravaginal probiotics that contain *L. rhamnosus* GR-1 and *L. reuteri* RC-14 may be used for the prevention of recurrent UTIs, either once or twice weekly for prophylaxis.

The daily use of the oral agents with strains GR-1 and RC-14 may restore the vaginal lactobacilli. These lactobacilli compete with urogenital pathogens and prevent bacterial vaginosis, a condition that increases the risk of UTIs.

There is evidence to suggest that cranberry (*Vaccinium macrocarpon*) is useful in reducing the rate of lower UTIs in women. The daily consumption of cranberry giving a minimum of 36 mg/day of proanthocyanindin A (the active compound) is recommended.

Q47. Answer E

Q48. Answer D

Q49. Answer C

Q50. Answer B

Q51. Answer A

UTIs are common during pregnancy. Most women acquire bacteriuria before pregnancy, and 20%–40% of women with asymptomatic bacteriuria develop pyelonephritis during pregnancy.

In an asymptomatic pregnant woman, bacteriuria is considered significant if two consecutive voided urine specimens grow $>10^5$ cfu/mL of the same bacterial species on quantitative culture; or a single catheterised specimen grows $>10^5$ cfu/mL of a uropathogen.

Pregnant women should be screened for bacteriuria during the first trimester and should be treated with antimicrobial therapy. Urine cultures should be obtained soon after completion of therapy for asymptomatic bacteriuria and symptomatic UTI in pregnancy.

Q52. Answer E

Q53. Answer D

Q54. Answer C

Q55. Answer B

Q56. Answer A

Epididymitis usually causes acute pain and swelling unilaterally. Chronic symptoms may develop in up to 15% of acute epididymitis cases. Acute epididymitis in young males is usually associated with sexual activity.

The most common type of orchitis, mumps orchitis, develops in 20%–30% of post-pubertal patients undergoing mumps infection. The incidence depends upon the vaccination status of the population.

Complications of epididymo-orchitis include abscess formation, testicular infarction, testicular atrophy, the development of chronic epididymal induration and infertility.

Epididymitis caused by sexually transmitted organisms occurs mainly in sexually active males aged < 35 years. The microbiological aetiology of epididymitis can usually be determined by examination of a Gram stain of a urethral smear and/or an MSU for the detection of Gram-negative bacteriuria. *C. trachomatis* will be isolated in approximately two-thirds of these patients.

Antimicrobials should be selected on the likely aetiology; in young, sexually active men *C. trachomatis* is usually causative and in older men with BPH or other urinary symptoms the most common uropathogens are involved. However, prior to antimicrobial therapy, a urethral swab and MSU should be obtained for further microbiological investigation. Fluoroquinolones, preferably those with activity against *C. trachomatis* (e.g., ofloxacin and levofloxacin), should be the drugs of first choice, because of their broad antibacterial spectra and their favourable penetration into the tissues of the urogenital tract. In cases caused by *C. trachomatis* treatment should also be considered with doxycycline, 200 mg/day, for a total treatment period of at least 2 weeks. In these the sexual partner should also be treated.

Q57. Answer F

Q58. Answer B

Q59. Answer C

Q60. Answer D

Q61. Answer A

It is estimated that infection *Mycobacterium tuberculosis* affects up to a third of the world's population. Genito-urinary tuberculosis is not common and is a severe form of extra-pulmonary tuberculosis. The diagnosis of genito-urinary tuberculosis is made based on culture studies by isolation of the causative organism. Drug treatment is the first line therapy with combination antibiotics for 6 months effective in most patients.

Xanthogranulomatous pyelonephritis (XGP), is a rare, serious, chronic inflammatory disorder of the kidney characterised by a destructive mass that invades the renal parenchyma. XGP is most commonly associated with *Proteus* or *Escherichia coli* infection, however *Pseudomonas* species have also been implicated. Pathologically, XGP is characterised by lipid-laden foamy macrophages. XGP may share many characteristics with renal tumours in terms of its radiographic appearance and its ability to involve adjacent structures or organs. XGP is often associated with urinary tract obstruction, infection, stones, diabetes, and an immuno-compromised state.

The treatment of severe XGP is almost universally surgical removal and can pose a formidable challenge to the surgeon. Most cases of XGP are unilateral and diffuse. The overall prognosis for XGP is good. Death from this entity is exceedingly rare, although morbidity is substantial.

Malakoplakia is a rare inflammatory condition which commonly presents as a papule, plaque or ulceration that usually affects the genito-urinary tract. Microscopically it is characterised by the presence of foamy histiocytes with basophilic inclusions called Michaelis-Gutmann bodies and usually involves gram-negative bacteria. Malakoplakia is thought to result from the insufficient killing of bacteria by macrophages and the partially digested bacteria therefore accumulate in macrophages and lead to a deposition of iron and calcium. The impairment of bactericidal activity manifests itself as the formation of an ulcer, plaque or papule. It is associated with patients with a history of immunosuppression due to lymphoma, diabetes mellitus, renal transplantation, or because of long-term therapy with systemic corticosteroids.

Emphysematous pyelonephritis (EPN) is a severe infection of the renal parenchyma that causes gas accumulation in the tissues. EPN is common in persons with diabetes, often has a fulminating course, and can be fatal if not recognised and treated promptly. The typical presenting features of EPN commonly include fever, abdominal or flank pain, nausea and vomiting, and acute renal impairment with confusion state.

Computed tomography (CT) scanning is the definitive imaging test for EPN. CT may show the gas patterns that are streaky, streaky and mottled, or streaky and bubbly, a rim-like or crescent-shaped gas collection in the perinephric area with or without a stone in the collecting system.

Early treatment is usually conservative with fluid resuscitation, systemic antibiotics, relief of obstruction with percutaneous drainage or stent placement and control of diabetes, if present. A nephrectomy may be required if there is no improvement after a drainage or failed drainage or when there is severe disease with high risk factors (the presence of more than two risk factors (e.g., thrombocytopenia, elevated serum creatinine, altered sensorium and shock).

REFERENCES

1. Bauer HW, Alloussi S, Egger G, Blumlein HM, Cozma G, Schulman CC. A long-term, multicenter, double-blind study of an *Escherichia coli* extract (OM-89) in female patients with recurrent urinary tract infections. *Eur Urol* 2005: **47**(4): 542–548.
2. Cribby S, Taylor M, Reid G. Vaginal microbiota and the use of probiotics. *Interdiscip Perspect Infect Dis* 2008: **2008**: 256490. doi:10.1155/2008/256490
3. Foo LY, Lu Y, Howell AB, Vorsa N. The structure of cranberry proanthocyanidins which inhibit adherence of uropathogenic P-fimbriated *Escherichia coli* in vitro. *Phytochemistry* 2000: **54**(2): 173–181.
4. Winberg J. P-fimbriae, bacterial adhesion, and pyelonephritis. *Arch Dis Child* 1984: **59**(2): 180–184.
5. Naber KG, Schito G, Botto H, Palou J, Mazzei T. Surveillance study in Europe and Brazil on clinical aspects and Antimicrobial Resistance Epidemiology in Females with Cystitis (ARESC): Implications for empiric therapy. *Eur Urol* 2008: **54**(5): 1164–1175.
6. Kramer G, Klingler HC, Steiner GE. Role of bacteria in the development of kidney stones. *Curr Opin Urol* 2000: **10**(1): 35–38.
7. Abrahams HM, Stoller ML. Infection and urinary stones. *Curr Opin Urol* 2003: **13**(1): 63–67.

CHAPTER 18: PAEDIATRIC UROLOGY

Jemma Hale and Arash K. Taghizadeh

MCQs

Q1. Which of the following investigations has the lowest radiation dose?
- A. Magnetic resonance urography (MRU)
- B. Plain abdominal X-ray
- C. MAG3 renogram
- D. DMSA renogram
- E. CT KUB

Q2. Which of these statements is CORRECT regarding religious circumcision?
- A. Consent for surgery from the mother is sufficient.
- B. The father can provide consent only if he is married to the boy's mother.
- C. Performing circumcision may be the least dangerous option.
- D. Where there is significant co-morbidity, counselling by a religious leader (e.g., priest) will have no value.
- E. Paediatric cardiology reassurance is required when the child has congenital heart disease.

Q3. Regarding undescended testis, which is the first step to be affected by the testis not having descended into the scrotum?
- A. Neonatal gonocyte
- B. Adult dark spermatogonia
- C. Adult pale spermatogonia
- D. Primary spermatocyte
- E. Spermatid

Q4. An 8-year-old boy presents with an inguinal testis. Which of the following is not true?
- A. The most likely explanation is that his undescended testis was missed on post-natal checks.
- B. Orchidopexy will not affect his risk of developing testicular malignancy.
- C. There is a possibility that his testis may descend spontaneously into his scrotum.
- D. An inguinal testis is at higher subsequent risk of undergoing torsion.
- E. If orchidopexy is performed an important step is the dissection and division of the processus vaginalis.

Q5. Which of the following are not associated with urinary incontinence in a child?
- A. Urinary flow rate indicating an overactive bladder
- B. Flattened buttocks
- C. Residual volume of 15 mL in a 5-year-old
- D. Faecal incontinence
- E. Inadequate leg abduction during voiding

Q6. Which of the following is not related to increased risk of nephroblastoma?
- A. Abnormality of chromosome 11 q
- B. Beckwith-Wiedemann syndrome
- C. Denys–Drash syndrome
- D. WAGR syndrome
- E. Perlman syndrome

Q7. Which of the following is not present at the presentation of a child with bladder exstrophy?
- A. Umbilicus adjacent to bladder plate
- B. Short length of intramural ureter entering the bladder plate
- C. Pubic diastasis
- D. Renal pelvicalyceal dilation
- E. Anterior anus

Q8. Which of these do not occur in a child with a disorder of sexual differentiation?
A. 21 α hydroxylase deficiency is associated with 46XX karyotype.
B. Androgen insensitivity syndrome is associated with 46XY karyotype.
C. 5α reductase deficiency is associated with 46XY karyotype.
D. Gondal dysgenesis is associated with 46XY karyotype.
E. Ovarian dysgenesis is associated with 45XO karyotype.

Q9. Which of the following is not true, with respect to myelomeningocele?
A. A low detrusor leak point pressure is associated with a worse outcome for the upper tracts.
B. Botulinum toxin A is not used children.
C. Tolterodine is not suitable for children.
D. Urethral intermittent catheterisation is rarely useful in children.
E. Ventriculoperitoneal shunt is a contraindication to ileocystoplasty.

EMQs

Q10–16. Investigation of renal tract abnormality
A. Serum creatinine
B. Renal ultrasound
C. MAG3
D. Micturating cystourethrogram
E. DMSA
F. Ultrasound scan of the spine
G. MRI scan of the spine
H. IVU
I. MRU

For each of the following clinical scenarios, which of the above would be the most appropriate investigation?

Q10. Newborn boy with antenatally detected bilateral pelvicalyceal and ureteric dilation with oligohydramnios.

Q11. A 2-month-old boy with antenatally detected bilateral pelvicalyceal and ureteric dilation. MCUG demonstrated a normal urethra, abnormal bladder and bilateral severe VUR.

Q12. A 3-month-old boy with antenatal unilateral hydronephrosis, persisting severe pelvicalyceal dilation but no ureteric dilatation.

Q13. A 3-month-old girl with antenatally unilateral hydronephrosis. Repeat ultrasound scan shows significant pelvicalyceal and ureteric dilatation. There is no reflux on MCUG.

Q14. A 9-month-old boy who presented with a pyrexial urinary tract infection aged 3 weeks. MCUG indicates primary unilateral VUR.

Q15. A 9-month-old boy who presented with a pyrexial urinary tract infection aged 3 weeks. MCUG indicates primary bilateral VUR.

Q16. A 5-year-old girl with primary continuous urinary incontinence. Ultrasound scan and DMSA are normal.

Q17–23. Embryology of the urinary tract
A. Mesonephric duct
B. Paramesonephric duct
C. Urogenital sinus
D. Metanephros
E. Mesonephros
F. Genital tubercle
G. Ureteric bud
H. Gubernaculum
I. Rathke's fold
J. Allantois

For each of the following anatomical structures described below, please give the correct embryological origin, from the list above.

Q17. Seminal vesicle

Q18. Utriculus

Q19. Epididymis

Q20. Ureteric bud

Q21. Urachal cyst

Q22. Gartner's cyst

Q23. Glomerulus

Q24–29. Hypospadias
  A. Meatal advancement glanuloplasty incorporated (MAGPI)
  B. Matthieu repair
  C. Snodgrass repair
  D. Two-stage repair
  E. Modified circumcision
  F. Foreskin repair
  G. Nesbitt repair
  H. Duckett repair
  I. De-gloving of the penis

For each of the operative descriptions below, please choose the correct description of hypospadias repair, from the list above.

Q24. Longitudinal midline incision of the urethral plate to facilitate tubularisation

Q25. Transverse urethral meatus

Q26. The most frequently used technique to correct the curvature of the penis

Q27. Regression of the urethral meatus

Q28. Foreskin used as a flap

Q29. Foreskin used as a graft

Q30–35. Surgical treatment options
  A. Careful medical management
  B. Supra-pubic catheter
  C. Vesicostomy
  D. Ureteric re-implant
  E. Ureterostomy
  F. Balloon dilation
  G. Pyelostomy
  H. Nephrostomy
  I. Endoscopic treatment of vesicoureteric reflux

For each of the following clinical scenarios listed below, please choose the most appropriate treatment option from the options listed above.

Q30. A 2 kg baby has a confirmed diagnosis of posterior urethral valves is managed with a urethral catheter because he is too small for cystoscopy and valve resection. On ultrasound he appears to have a non-dilated kidney with normal cortico-medullary differentiation on one side, and a small kidney with a very dilated pelvicalycaeal system and ureter on the other side but with no vesicoureteric reflux. He has had a second urinary tract infection since being managed with a urethral catheter.

Q31. An 18-month-old girl with a second pyrexial urinary tract infection, despite prophylactic antibiotics, and known to have Grade V vesicoureteric reflux.

Q32. A 6-month-old boy with a second urinary tract infection since being diagnosed with bilateral grade V primary vesicoureteric reflux.

Q33. A 4-month-old presents with a urinary tract infection. She has unilateral marked pelvicalyceal and ureteric dilatation, associated with 38% function, impaired drainage on MAG3 and no reflux on micturating cystogram.

Q34. A 9-month-old boy has posterior urethral valves which have been resected. His estimated glomerular filtration rate is 20 mL/min/1.73. He has a solitary kidney with gross peliv-calyceal dilation. He has severe reflux into his upper tract through a very tortuous ureter. He continues to have recurrent severe urinary tract infections.

Q35. A 9-month-old girl presents with her first pyrexial urinary tract infection. She has unilateral grade III reflux.

Q36–39. Multisystem disorders and syndromes
    A. Posterior urethral valve
    B. Sacral agenesis
    C. Cloaca
    D. Cloacal exstrophy
    E. Spinal dysraphism
    F. Anorectal malformation
    G. VACTERL
    H. Severe constipation

For the statements listed below, which of the clinical conditions listed above is the most appropriate?

Q36. Not associated with abnormal bowel function

Q37. Characteristically associated with a maternal history of diabetes mellitus

Q38. Affects only girls

Q39. Is least likely to be associated with a spinal abnormality

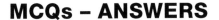

MCQs – ANSWERS

Q1. Answer B

The approximate radiation burden for these investigations:

- MRU involves no radiation. However, the need to lie still during the investigation limits the test without general anaesthesia to those who infants less than 3 months old ('feed and wrap') and children above about 11 years.

- MAG3: 0.20–0.38 mSv (mSv = milli Sievert)

- DMSA: This is approximately 1 mSv/examination regardless of the age of the child (providing that the dose is adapted according to body surface). The radioactive tracer is taken up and binds to the proximal convoluted tubules and retained there with the image taken after 2–3 hours.

- Plain abdominal x-ray dose in a child 1.0 mSv.

- CT KUB: abdomen/pelvis child 10 mSv. Low-dose CT can achieve doses of less than 3.5 mSv, and ultra-low-dose CT of less than 1.9 mSv.

Q2. Answer C

This is a question about consent and ethics. The starting point is that the parents are requesting a surgical procedure that does not carry a clinical benefit. The BMA and GMC recommend that the consent of both parents should be obtained for a procedure that is non-therapeutic and 'important and irreversible.' Previously, fathers that were not married to the mother did not have parental responsibility and so were unable to give consent for surgical procedures. However, the law has changed. For children born after 1 December 2003, if their father's name appears on the birth certificate, then the father does have parental responsibility. This does not apply to children born before this date. It should be remembered that grandparents, close family friends, etc cannot provide informed consent for a child's surgery. Conversely a child with sufficient capacity may provide their own consent. The problems around religious circumcision come to a focus where the child has significant co-morbidity (e.g., cardiac disease or coagulopathy). Parents are often strongly motivated to have circumcision performed for cultural reasons. Where the child has significant co-morbidity these motivations should be carefully explored with the parents. Surgical circumcision does carry risk, but circumcision performed outside of a hospital in less controlled settings is a far less satisfactory option. Parents who are denied a hospital circumcision may proceed to arrange a circumcision in the community. It can be very helpful for the parent to meet and have a discussion with the religious leader from their religion (e.g., priest). The advice is often given that their religion discourages circumcision if it endangers the child. In my practice I also recommend that the parents have a discussion with an appropriate anaesthetist who is better able to counsel about anaesthetic risks in the face of significant cardiac or respiratory disease. For example, a cardiac anaesthetist is better placed to counsel about anaesthesia risk than a paediatric cardiologist where there is congenital heart disease.

Q3. Answer A

The transition from neonatal gonocyte to adult dark spermatogonia takes place at 3–12 months in humans. Between the first and fourth years of life the spermatogonia differentiate into B-spermatogonia, and then primary spermatocytes. These then remain quiescent until puberty triggers spermatogenesis. The transformation of the neonatal gonocyte into the adult dark spermatogonia appears to be a crucial stage. It seems to be dependent on the environment of these cells being at 33°C. Failure of the testicle to descend into the scrotum keeps the testis at 37°C and so adversely affects this stage. Transformation from neonatal gonocyte to adult dark spermatogonia includes a reduction in the number of these cells probably reflecting apoptosis of abnormal cells. Failure of the testicle to descend by this stage will result in reduced sperm production but also less removal of abnormal cells probably contributing to increased risk of subsequent malignant transformation. Recognition that this stage takes place quite early has resulted in the British Association of Paediatric Urologist recommending in 2011 earlier orchidopexy. Ideally orchidopexy should be performed between 3–6 months; however, 6–12 months is acceptable.

Q4. Answer A

There had previously been an assumption that boys presenting at this late age with an undescended testis had previously had this finding missed at previous checks. However this age group represent a significant proportion of boys undergoing orchidopexy. At post-natal checks, where there is little adipose, the cremasteric reflex is weak and the testes are prominent, identifying undescended testes is relatively easy. It was realised from carefully documented examinations that testes that had previously been identified in the scrotum had subsequently ascended.

The mechanism for testicular ascent is not clear. One possibility is the presence of a processus vaginalis remnant, which because of a relatively slower rate of growth than the rest of the child would drag the testis up as the inguinal canal lengthened. Alternatively, it is possible that a proportion of these boys originally had retractile testes an overactive cremaster had permanently brought these testes up.

In the Netherlands and Scandinavia ascending testes are managed expectantly as about half will descend spontaneously. However the UK practice (according to the 2011 consensus from the British Association of Paediatric Urologists) is to offer surgery. It is not clear what effect there will be on the testis and on sperm production if the testis is left in the groin waiting for puberty. There is evidence that performing orchidopexy before puberty may halve the risk of malignancy for undescended testes. Although it is not clear that ascended testes are at increased risk of malignancy, it can be difficult in practice to distinguish an ascended from a missed undescended testis.

Q5. Answer C

A 'tower' shaped flow rate can give a useful indication of an overactive bladder. The appearance of flattened buttocks is characteristic of sacral agenesis and neuropathic bladder.

The ICCS definition of abnormal residual volume a little difficult to remember. For children aged 4–6 years, the residual volume is abnormal if on *repeated measures* it is more than 20 mL or more than 10% of bladder capacity (bladder capacity = voided volume + residual volume). For children who are 7–12 years repeated measured residual of more than 10 mL, or 6% of bladder capacity are abnormal.

If a history of faecal incontinence is volunteered then more careful evaluation is required. Most commonly faecal incontinence is a manifestation of constipation. Assessment of a child with constipation would include asking how often the child opens their bowels, whether there is associated pain or blood, examination of the abdomen for palpable stool and checking for spinal abnormality. A bowel diary kept over a week can be useful including comparison against the Bristol stool chart. Treatment of constipation will frequently result in resolution of urinary symptoms. However, faecal leaking may be a manifestation of neuropathic bladder and bowel. It is possible however that faecal leaking may be related to spinal abnormality. It is important that this is considered, other symptoms and signs of abnormality sought, and if there is adequate concern, spinal imaging arranged.

Vaginal reflux is a cause of post-micturition wetting in girls. It is effectively treated by abducting the legs widely during voiding.

Q6. Answer A

Nephroblastoma, or Wilms' tumour, characteristically presents as a painless mass in an otherwise well pre-school child. In the UK, after staging imaging the diagnosis is made with biopsy. Treatment begins with chemotherapy, and is then followed by surgery. Further chemotherapy or radiotherapy may then follow.

The WT1 gene, predisposing to the Wilms' tumour, lies on chromosome 11p13. Other genes predisposing to Wilms' tumours have also been identified at 11p15 and 16q.

Beckwith–Wiedemann syndrome is characterised by macroglossia, macrosomia, visceromegaly and midline abdominal wall defect such as omphalocele or exomphalos. It is associated with a significantly increased risk of developing Wilms' tumour.

Perlman syndrome is another overgrowth syndrome associated with polyhydramnios during pregnancy, macrocephaly, macrosomia, visceromegaly and an increased risk for Wilms' tumour.

In Denys–Drash syndrome, the presence of nephropathy (mesangial sclerosis) and gonadal dysgenesis is associated with the development of Wilms' tumour.

WAGR syndrome is characterised by increased predisposition to Wilms' tumour, aniridia, genitourinary anomalies (typical tumours of the ovaries or testes) and 'mental retardation'.

Q7. Answer D

The abnormalities seen in bladder exstrophy represent a failure of development of the lower abdominal wall; possibly because of the failure of mesoderm to migrate into the cloacal membrane. In classic bladder exstrophy the abnormalities seen all follow from this failure. The bladder lies open and exposed as a bladder plate. The umbilicus lies immediately adjacent to the bladder plate. When the bladder plate is mobilised for closure the umbilicus becomes ischaemic and is subsequently lost. The ureters do not enter the bladder obliquely and there is an increased tendency to subsequent vesicoureteric reflux. There is diastasis of the pubic rami, (i.e., they fail to meet in the midline). The lower abdominal wall demonstrates a series of characteristic features: the rectus muscle divaricates inferiorly, the umbilicus is sited rather low, and the perineum is foreshortened resulting in a slightly anterior anus. The separated pubic rami result in the bony attachments of the corpora cavernosa being widely separated. This contributes to a rather short and wide penis in boys, and a bifid clitoris in girls.

In contrast to cloacal exstrophy, there tend not to be other associated anomalies in classic bladder exstrophy, (i.e., there is no increased association with developmental problems, cardiac or spinal disease).

Although bladder exstrophy is a devastating anomaly of the lower urinary tract, the upper urinary tract is not usually affected at presentation. Closure of the abdominal wall and bladder are difficult. To achieve urinary continence, some mechanism to control the bladder outlet needs to be surgically created, as well as ensuring that the bladder has adequate storage. One of the most common ways of controlling the bladder outlet is to create a fixed resistance that then has to be overcome during voiding. Care of these complex patients is performed in specialist centres where the goal of urinary continence is perused without jeopardising the upper tracts.

Q8. Answer E

For those that do not practice in this area, disorders of sexual differentiation (DSD) can prove difficult to understand. It would seem unfair that someone taking the FRCS(Urol) would have a detailed knowledge of the classification of these conditions. A few basic principles will be outlined.

A very simplified account of the embryology of differentiation follows. The foetus will develop by default into a female. The mesonephric duct (precursors of uterus and upper vagina) are initially present in both males and females. Secretion of Müllerian Inhibiting Substance (MIS) from the Sertoli cells from 7 weeks will cause regression of the mesonephric duct structures in boys. Androgens, and especially dihydroxy-testosterone are responsible for the development of the external genitals in males.

A good starting point for classifying DSD is the karyotype. Those with 46XX who have DSD will be over-virilised; those with 46XY who have DSD will be under-virilised. This will be further complicated by mosaic karyotype patterns.

The next consideration is the development of the gonads. Where gonads have formed abnormally there is gonadal dysgenesis. This may be complete or partial. It may result in streak gonads or in an ovo-testis combination.

Then next consideration is whether there is an abnormality in the synthesis of the sex-hormone or their receptor. In congenital adrenal hyperplasia, the production of cortisol and aldosterone is disrupted triggering over production of ACTH which then stimulates overproduction of androgenic precursors resulting in over virilisation of girls. Androgen receptor insensitivity and 5α reductase deficiency will on the other hand result in under-virilised boys.

Ovarian dysgenesis syndrome is also known as Turner's syndrome. Dysgenetic streak ovaries are present but in the absence of a Y chromosome there is no cause for ambiguity about the appearance of the genitals.

Q9. Answer A

The detrusor leak point pressure is the lowest pressure at which leaking occurs without detrusor contraction or rise in abdominal pressure. Pressures over 40 cm of water are associated with increased risk of upper tract damage.

Poor bladder emptying is most reliably managed with urethral intermittent catheterisation. This can be very daunting for the patient and the parents. However a good clinical nurse specialist can be surprisingly successful in even the most anxious children. Teaching clean intermittent catheterisation to the parents of all infants with myelomeningocele within the first year will avoid the problems of having to teach an older and more reluctant child.

The first line treatment of detrusor over-activity is anti-muscarinic medication. Although oxybutynin is probably the most commonly used, tolterodine is also frequently effective.

Botulinum toxin is increasingly being used in the management of neurogenic detrusor over-activity. Treatment is administered under general anaesthesia, and requires repeating. It is best reserved for those who do not tolerate or respond to anti-muscarinics.

Ileocystoplasty is a very effective treatment of unsafe bladder storage. It is a significant undertaking. Those treated this way will have increase urinary mucus, and face increased risk of infection, stones, alkalosis, Vitamin B_{12} deficiency, bladder rupture and possibly malignancy. Although there is a risk of infection of ventriculoperitoneal shunt, this is not a contraindication to ileocystoplasty.

EMQs – ANSWERS

Q10. Answer D

Q11. Answer F

Q12. Answer C

Q13. Answer C

Q14. Answer E

Q15. Answer A

Q16. Answer I

There is no absolute rule correct way to investigate renal tract anomalies but a guideline is provided below.

The most common causes of hydronephrosis are listed below. The additional comments are not diagnostic criteria but provide the first thread to follow when trying to diagnose the underlying anomaly. Hydronephrosis can occur without functional problems such as obstruction or reflux.

PUJ obstruction	Pelvicalyceal dilation only
VUJ obstruction	Pelvicalyceal and ureteric dilation
Vesicoureteric reflux	Pelvicalyceal and ureteric dilation
Posterior urethral valves	Bilateral pelvicalyceal dilation (with or without ureteric dilation) in a boy.
Other things to consider	Neuropathic bladder Complex anomalies such as ectopic ureters persistent cloaca, urogenital sinus

The investigations are used for answering specific questions.

Renal US scan

In the first week of life when the child is relatively dehydrated, an ultrasound scan can underestimate the degree of hydronephrosis. If such an early scan shows an improvement compared to the prenatal scans, this should not provide reassurance that things have improved.

MAG3

Indicates the relative split function of the kidney. Because it generates dynamic pictures it will identify impaired renal drainage. It should be used where upper tract obstruction is suspected.

MCUG – micturating cystourethrogram

Requires catheter insertion and hence is a very invasive test for a child especially after one year of age. Good urethral views in boys are required to establish or exclude the presence of posterior urethral valves. It can also indicate bladder abnormality such as enlargement or trabeculation. It demonstrates the anatomy of reflux.

DMSA

Like a MAG3 scan, it provides split function. A DMSA scan provides a static picture which is of higher resolution than a MAG3. It is therefore very useful for identifying areas of defective renal cortical function. When it is done acutely it can be used to support a diagnosis of pyelonephritis. If the question is to identify the presence of renal scarring following pyelonephritis, then the DMSA scan should be postponed for 6 months after the acute episode.

Ultrasound scan of the spine

Before the spine ossifies, ultrasound can be used to identify abnormalities of the spinal cord. It is less valuable after three months of age when the bones calcify. It is a very useful test to do in babies in whom a neuropathic bladder is suspected.

MRI scan of the spine

Gives the most detailed information about spinal cord abnormalities. Young children will often require general anaesthetic or sedation.

IVU

Very rarely performed in children; other modalities are much more useful because it is so infrequently performed it is difficult to maintain the experience to generate good images. There is little role for it outside a specialist unit and even then it is usually used to answer very specific questions.

MRU

With correct sequences performed in experienced hands, MRU can delineate complex renal tract anatomy. However it often requires a general anaesthetic in a younger child.

If posterior urethral valves are the primary concern, the renal function of this child is likely to be poor but a creatinine may not give an accurate indication of this for a few days. The child requires bladder drainage, fluid management and a diagnostic test (i.e., an MCUG). With a normal urethra but abnormal bladder and upper tracts there is the possibility of a neuropathic bladder. In early life it is easy to look for spinal abnormalities with an US scan. If the concern is PUJ obstruction, a MAG3 gives the most useful information. Ureteric dilatation without reflux raises the possibility of congenital obstruction such as VUJ obstruction. Again, a MAG3 gives the most useful information. Where there is unilateral renal disease, this is unlikely to be reflected in the creatinine. When both kidneys are affected by disease it is more important to know the overall renal function before knowing whether there is scarring. Clinically, if there is a suspicion that this girl has an ectopic ureter, with a normal renal ultrasound scan, it is unlikely that the ectopic ureter would have arisen from a duplex kidney. An ectopic ureter arising from a duplex kidney can arise from a very small and poorly functioning upper pole. This can be difficult to find on ultrasound scan and DMSA. Careful MRI sequences can identify an otherwise cryptic duplex kidney.

Q17. Answer A

Q18. Answer A

Q19. Answer A

Q20. Answer A

Q21. Answer J

Q22. Answer A

Q23. Answer D

The Mesonephric (Wolffian) duct gives rise to most of the structures in the male genital tract which includes: ejaculatory ducts, seminal vesicles, vas deferens, epididymii. In females the mesonephric duct remnants include the epoöphoron, paraoöphoron and Gartner's cyst. In addition and importantly, in males and females, it gives rise to the ureteric bud which gives rise to the ureter, renal pelvis, major calyces, minor calyces and collecting ducts. The very end of the mesonephric duct gives rise to the trigone.

The gubernaculum begins as mesenchymal tissue from the lower pole of the testes and extends into what becomes the scrotum. A pouch of peritoneum extends into the gubernaculum to form the processes vaginalis which then involute behind the testis as it descends into the scrotum.

The paramesonephric (Müllerian) duct gives rise to most of the structures in the female genital tract: the uterus, Fallopian tubes and upper two thirds of the vagina. The lower third of the vagina and the vaginal vestibule originates from the urogenital sinus. Persistence of the paramesonephric duct in males may result in the presence of a utriculus, which is a midline cystic structure inserting into the verumontanum of the urethra. In boys, it can also give rise to a testicular appendix.

The kidney is formed after the ureteric bud grows into the metanephros by process of reciprocal induction. Urine production in the foetus begins around 10 weeks. The metanephros gives rise to the glomeruli, convoluted tubules and loop of Henle.

The urogenital sinus gives rise to the bladder and the urethra in females. In males the urogenital sinus accounts for the bladder and the posterior urethra. The penile urethra is formed by fusion of the genital folds and canalisation of the tip of the glans.

The genital tubercle gives rise to the clitoris in females and the penis in boys.

The prostate is formed by reciprocal induction of the urogenital sinus and adjacent mesenchyme.

The cloaca is a primitive cavity, which ultimately separates into the rectum and urogenital sinus. Rathke's folds originate laterally and meet in the midline helping to separate the cloaca into these two cavities.

The Allantois is a cavity that communicates with the urogenital sinus. Persistence of this communication gives rise to urachal remnants, for example, urachal sinus, fistula or cysts.

Q24. Answer C

Q25. Answer B

Q26. Answer I

Q27. Answer A

Q28. Answer H

Q29. Answer D

The great variety of hypospadias repair indicates that each has its shortcomings. For mild or glanular hypospadias the author would perform a modified circumcision or foreskin reconstruction. For less mild distal hypospadias, Snodgrass (tubularised incised plate) repair gives acceptable results. For more proximal hypospadias or where there is severe curvature, a two-stage repair using inner prepuce as a graft is used.

A MAGPI hypospadias repair can be used for mild hypospadias but tends to give an unsightly meatus. The Matthieu repair uses a flap of ventral shaft skin to complete the urethral tube but results in a transverse meatus. Duckett described using a flap of prepucial skin to repair the urethra; in the longer term this often results in a urethra that becomes excessively dilated.

Q30. Answer H

Q31. Answer D

Q32. Answer C

Q33. Answer F

Q34. Answer G

Q35. Answer A

These are all difficult paediatric urology problems. It is perhaps unfair to offer solutions in an MCQ format as there is often no absolute or single correct answer. It is hoped that the explanations below will provide some insight into some of the principles that inform decision making in paediatric urology.

The first step in preventing urinary tract infection is good medical management. This includes maintaining a good fluid intake, regular bladder emptying, control of constipation and consideration of prophylactic antibiotics. When medical management doesn't work, then surgery should be considered.

One of the most important considerations is function. This overrides considerations about appearance and anatomy. For example, upper tract dilation with sluggish drainage on MAG3 is less of a concern where there are a series of renograms over several years showing that kidney is maintaining its function. However similar drainage on renography has a very different interpretation where there are either symptoms, infection or reduced function in that kidney.

The goal is ensuring good urinary drainage. Good urinary drainage protects against symptoms, infection and declining function. This is the central principle that all urologists apply to their daily practice. It is the basis of advice given to patients with recurrent infections to drink well and void regularly. It is why intermittent catheterisation (perhaps counter intuitively) reduces the risk of the patients who perform it. It is why urinary tract stomas reduce infection risk despite opening the urinary tract to the skin.

Indwelling catheters achieve drainage but quickly become colonised by bacteria and so are not an ideal long term solution. There is no advantage of supra-pubic over urethral catheterisation in this respect. In an infant it is relatively easy to bring any part of the urinary tract to the surface. The stoma is usually managed without a bag; often a folded nappy is sufficient to control the urinary efflux.

A final principle is that urinary tract obstruction can be difficult to identify. A useful definition of obstruction is that it is an impairment in urinary flow that if untreated would cause a decline in renal function. In the light of this definition, renograms do not provide this level of prediction and a clinician must be very wary of MAG3 reports that unequivocally identify or exclude obstruction.

Boys with posterior urethral valves can develop a secondary VUJ obstruction after their bladder is drained. There thick-walled bladder pinches down on the distal ureter. This is usually self-limiting and will resolve. However, the boy described appears to have infection problems as a result of impaired drainage across his VUJ. He is too young for a MAG3. A nephrostomy will allow drainage and allow subsequent nephrostogram.

Endoscopic treatment of high-grade reflux can be disappointing; the success rate the treating grade V VUR is a little more than 50%. Ureteric reimplantation is a reasonable choice for severe reflux.

It is considered that ureteric reimplantation in infants under a year of age should be avoided. Severe bilateral 'primary' reflux in a boy is often associated with coexisting abnormal bladder function. This boy may have significant incomplete bladder emptying. Improving his bladder drainage is likely to reduce risk of urinary infection. This may include clean intermittent catheterisation or these are customary.

The 4-month-old girl with impaired drainage of her dilated kidney and ureter is likely to have poor drainage across her VUJ. She is too small to have ureteric reimplantation. She may respond to balloon dilation and stenting of her VUJ.

The boy with posterior urethral valves has a reduced renal function and the priority is to preserve the little function he has. Bringing his renal pelvis out as stoma may reduce his infection risk by improving urine drainage and diverting it away from his slow draining ureter.

Q36. Answer A

Q37. Answer B

Q38. Answer C

Q39. Answer A

Many of these conditions are infrequently seen in adult urology clinics; however, all will impact the urinary tract.

Posterior urethral valves occur as a congenital obstruction of the bladder outflow. All subsequent problems in a boy with posterior urethral valves follow from the obstruction that is present during the development of the bladder and upper tract. Other systems (e.g., cardiac or nervous) are not affected.

Abnormal bladder function is seen in up to 40% of children with anorectal malformation. This may be directly because of the condition or the very frequent association with spinal abnormality. Persistent cloaca is a severe form of anorectal malformation seen in girls where the bladder, bowel and vagina converge and open onto the perineum as a single channel. The VACTERAL association includes the presence of vertebral, anorectal, cardiac, tracheo-oesophageal, renal and limb anomalies.

Maternal diabetes is a predisposing factor for sacral agenesis. In this condition, the nerve supply of the sacral segments is disrupted, resulting in a neuropathic bladder and bowel. The condition is characterised by flattened buttocks because of affected innervation of the gluteal muscles.

Constipation can be a significant aggravating factor for urinary symptoms. Effective treatment of constipation will often effectively treat urinary symptoms as well. It is however always worth considering the possibility of underlying spinal disease in children being managed for apparently functional urinary or bowel symptoms, if only to examine the back, buttocks and lower limbs.

Index

Note: Page numbers in italic and bold refer to figures and tables, respectively.